HERBAL THERAPY FOR WOMEN

Elisabeth Brooke qualified as a Medical Herbalist with the National Institute of Medical Herbalists in 1980 and opened and runs a training clinic for herbal students in London. She also has a private practice in London and teaches and lectures worldwide.

For more information and contact details, please visit www.elisabethbrooke.com

HERBAL
THERAPY
FOR
WOMEN

Elisabeth Brooke

First published in 1992 by Thorsons, an imprint of HarperCollins.

This edition published 2018 by

Aeon Books Ltd
12 New College Parade
Finchley Road
London NW3 5EP

British Library Cataloguing in Publication Data

A C.I.P. for this book is available from the British Library

ISBN-13: 978-1-91159-724-7

www.aeonbooks.co.uk

Contents

Introduction

WHY HERBALISM?

ALTHOUGH HERBAL MEDICINE has been used for a very long time, it is only in recent years that the general public has become familiar with its existence. Increasingly disenchanted with orthodox methods of treatment, people are searching for a different approach to sickness and health. Potent chemical drugs with their dangerous side-effects and courses of treatment which often cause more problems than they cure, have all helped to persuade people to look again at the treatment of sickness and ask themselves if there is not another way.

One of the criticisms of orthodox medicine is that it treats the symptoms but not the cause of an illness. What does this mean? For example, if a woman has cystitis, she might undergo a course of treatment which clears the infection. Another woman might have repeated attacks of cystitis and take one treatment after another. The attacks may become more frequent or severe and either her body begins to build up a resistance to the treatment or side-effects such as thrush begin to appear.

Clearly, the first woman has found orthodox treatment helpful. The second woman is the type of case that arrives at my clinic. Since there is less emphasis on the causes of illness, the orthodox practitioner treating the second woman will probably continue trying one remedy after another, using stronger and stronger forms of treatment and possibly resorting to drastic kinds of surgery such as cautery. Other conventional practitioners might go into the more psychological aspects of her case to see whether there are emotional problems which are contributing factors. But apart from this, there would be little that orthodox medicine could offer. For this reason, the second woman might well seek out alternative forms of treatment.

I do not intend this to be a polemic against orthodox treatment, since it has its place in the scheme of things and is excellent for emergencies and certain kinds of surgery. However, in the treatment of chronic, long-lasting illnesses, orthodox treatment has little to offer in the way of a solution. This is why an increasing number of people are looking for alternatives to orthodox medicine.

So what does herbal medicine have to offer?

Let's go back to our two cases. In the first case, the herbal approach might seem to be similar. A short course of treatment would be prescribed, which would be designed to clear up the infection and build up the body's general resistance. In the second case, the treatment would be very different. A herbal practitioner would investigate the causes of an illness in far greater detail than would the orthodox practitioner. In looking for causes, the herbalist would want to discover the reasons for the illness and the category of complaint. Orthodox diagnosis might describe only one level of the illness, whereas an alternative practitioner would have several descriptions or explanations for the condition. Cystitis, for example, might be due to a chill in the bladder, in which case a gentle warming remedy would be called for. Alternatively, the infection could be caused by irritation and heat in the bladder and a soothing, cooling herb would be prescribed. Besides these two very different methods of treatment, the practitioner would also look at the general health of the body to check the circulation and the function of the lungs and heart. This would enable the practitioner to adjust any existing imbalances in the body which may have been contributing factors to the genesis of the illness. Lastly, the herbalist would prescribe a healing restorative tonic, which would gradually restore diseased tissues to a state of equilibrium and health.

So the approach to treatment is completely different. The patient is seen as a whole being and the symptom, cystitis, is viewed in the context of the whole person and the complicated interactions between the different parts of the body, and patient's physical and emotional states. Herbal treatment is aimed at gently aiding the immune system of the body to fight off infection as well as heal the damaged tissue. Because this is a lengthy process, herbal treatment is slow, gently re-balancing the body, healing in a gradual but sure fashion.

This approach is particularly important in the treatment of women's complaints. Over the years, they have developed into a speciality of mine for several reasons: firstly, as a woman I have a certain sympathy and interest in women and an understanding of their problems and preoccupations; secondly, and more importantly, because of my experience with women in a clinical setting.

The majority of my patients have been women; this might be because in general women consult their medical practitioners more than men, or because they are less satisfied with the treatment they receive from orthodox medical practitioners. It has certainly been my experience that gynaecologists and obstetricians often lack sensitivity when dealing with their women patients. I have heard countless stories of patients being ignored, ridiculed or not taken seriously, and more serious accounts of bullying and rough treatment at the hands of insensitive specialists. I have, at this point, to make it clear that it is not only male orthodox practitioners who are guilty on this score; women doctors and complementary medical workers of both sexes do not necessarily behave any better to their female patients. I do not want to look for scapegoats or to lay the blame at any one door, but to explain the value in looking at an alternative approach to the treatment of woman's diseases.

Although the woman's movement has done much to educate both professional and lay people, there is still an astonishing amount of ignorance about women's health and women's bodies. The mysterious and quixotic nature of women's physiology often defies rational understanding, and because woman's emotions are connected to their menstrual cycles and their relationship to fertility and childbearing, emotions run high. For these reasons, there exists a great deal of misunderstanding as to the real nature of women's experience. This needs to be coupled with the realization that modern medicine is no longer an art, but a science: by this I mean a logical linear understanding, or explanation of physical phenomena. This in itself is neither a good nor a bad thing, but given the nature of women's experience of their reproductive cycle, it is hardly adequate. Hormones are not simply miniscule amounts of potent chemicals which whizz around the bloodstream and have physical effects; they affect the mental, emotional and physical balance of the body in both subtle and gross ways. Any woman who is pregnant or premenstrual knows how fractional changes in her hormone levels drastically affect how she feels and behaves. Women often find themselves acting in most uncharacteristic ways, only to discover that their period has started the following day and hormonal changes have brought on this 'madness'.

As I hope I have explained in the chapter on common complaints, these hormonal shifts can be used for good or ill. Depending on the resources and the point of view of the woman, it can be a time of great creativity or awful emotional strain. This wide range of experience does not respond well to physical doses of synthetic hormones. Clearly, such a clash of experiences only leads to misunderstandings, impatience and intolerance on both sides. The women end up feeling that they are crazy or are imagining what they are feeling, and the doctors are intensely frustrated since there is very little that medical science can offer them; they feel that they are unable to help and tend to express this to the women concerned.

From my perspective, anyone treating women's ailments needs to have a good deal of understanding and sympathy for women as well as a wider perspective of their ailments. As practitioners, we also need to counter the implicit belief that what is normal or standard is masculine and what is abnormal is female. When we are pregnant we are healthy, not sick; menstruating women are not unclean, nor are they ill, but are performing a simple biological function; menopausal women are passing through another, equally important stage of life. Health workers need to be educated to appreciate and understand this point of view and to approach the treatment of women's complaints from a more sympathetic and gentle perspective.

The majority of women who arrived at my door came traumatized and often desperate. To them, I was the last chance. They were strong women who refused to put up with their crippling menstrual pain or debilitating pre-menstrual symptoms, and refused to follow the line of thinking that all this was 'Eve's curse'. Not all women have the time to search out a listening ear, or the money to pay for private treatment: for this reason, I wrote this book. I hope that the women who read it take heart and courage from its pages, are able to understand more about their bodies and the phases and cycles they go through and can use the sections containing practical information to help alleviate some of their health problems.

This was my intention in writing this book, and I hope that I have to some extent fulfilled my aims.

CAUTION

While in my professional opinion, all the herbs that I have discussed in the book can be taken safely, provided the doses I have recommended are followed and any contra-indications strictly adhered to, some people might have reactions to individual herbs which cannot be predicted by generalities. That is to say, each person is an individual and has his or her idiosyncracies which can only be predicted by a skilled practitioner.

Some of the herbs mentioned in this book, notably comfrey and bearberry have been found to have side effects in anecdotal experience and clinical trials.

If you are taking prescription drugs always tell your doctor if you want to use herbal prescriptions as well. Many people are worried about telling their doctors about using complementary therapies, for fear they might anger or upset them. This may have been the case several years ago and some doctors still remain hostile to complementary medicine. However, the majority of doctors are open-minded if not enthusiastic about alternative approaches.

Self-treatment is fine for simple ailments, but is not to be recommended for long-standing or chronic conditions. If you develop an illness and treat it with herbs and it has not cleared up after two weeks, seek professional advice.

It is, however, extremely dangerous suddenly to stop taking certain kinds of prescription drugs, especially barbiturates, tranquillizers, steroids and heart drugs. On no account should patients reduce the dosage of these remedies without medical supervision. Any complementary health practitioner who suggests this is going beyond his or her brief and his or her advice should not be followed.

PREGNANCY

I have not included a section on herbs for pregnancy because I feel it is unwise to self-prescribe at this time. Under individual herbs, mention is made of their use by practitioners for some complaints which might arise in pregnancy, but for safety's sake, always consult a herbalist for specialist advice. This includes herbal teas, the majority of which are safe and have no side-effects, but my belief is that it is wise to err on the side of caution and avoid anything – foods, drinks or medicine – which might harm the new life. The following herbs should never be taken during pregnancy: pennyroyal, myrrh, barberry, poke root, false unicorn root. If in doubt, contact a practitioner. Do not use herbal remedies during pregnancy without professional advice; especially during the first three months. Likewise, babies and children should only be treated with herbs under the supervision of a herbal health professional.

HOW TO FIND A PRACTITIONER

In the UK, anyone can set themselves up as an alternative practitioner without qualifications. The situation is different in other countries and is generally more strictly controlled. The best way to find a reliable practitioner is through personal recommendation; qualifications do give the public an assurance of a level of competence though they are never watertight, as the disciplinary council of the General Medical Council will testify. Ask your friends or the workers at the local health food store and of course, use common sense. If you trust and feel safe with a practitioner, he or she will be good for you; if you are doubtful, feel them to be unsympathetic or simply do not like the advice that they give you, find another one. Check whether the practitioner has treated similar conditions, and what their results were. Ask beforehand how long your treatment will last, and how long it is likely to take before you can expect to see any improvement in your illness. Also ask what the fees will be and whether there is a sliding scale or reduction for senior citizens or the unemployed. In London the fees are currently about £20-£30 per hour; in the provinces, slightly less. Don't allow the therapist to blame you for your illness; the genesis of illness is complicated and multi-faceted. It is facile and incorrect to assume we are 'guilty' in this respect. Lastly, miracles do occur, but most healing is a slow erratic process. Your co-operation as a patient is essential to any cure.

In the UK, qualified practitioners have the letters MNIMH after their names. The Council for Complementary and Alternative Medicine, 21 Portland Place, London W1, tel (071) 636 9545 has an information service and a register of complementary and alternative practitioners. In other countries, there are different governing bodies which can be contacted through libraries and health food stores.

AVAILABILITY OF HERBS

I have tried to keep the number of plants discussed as low as possible because I feel it is far more useful to know a few plants well than wade through endless unfamiliar names. With the exception of myrrh and ginger, all of the plants are to be found in Europe. Most of the herbs mentioned in this book can be obtained locally in health food stores in the UK, USA and Australia.

The following herbs are not indigenous to the Americas, but some may be imported: archangel; lady's mantle; lavender; melissa; vitex. These herbs are not found in Australia, but may be imported: archangel; lady's mantle; melissa; motherwort; squaw vine; false unicorn root.

1   *Practical Information*

THIS SECTION EXPLAINS in detail how to make your own herbal remedies. Although they may seem complicated, anyone who is a fair cook, or who knows her way around the kitchen will have no problem following the directions. For those who do not have the time to make their own preparations there are several alternatives. Herbal teas are available in most wholefood shops and can also be used, but to make them of medicinal strength, use two tea bags per cup. Herbal tinctures are also available; follow the dosage on the container, as with any herbal pills and tablets.

HOW TO COLLECT AND STORE HERBS, ROOTS AND SEEDS

Even the most confirmed city-dweller can collect his or her own herbs. People are often very surprised when I say this, considering the rising pollution levels in our towns and cities. Be sensible; don't pick your plants by the side of a motorway, nor near a factory belching out toxic waste. Bear in mind that in most cities there is a lot of waste ground, parkland, commons and back gardens. These places usually contain a wealth of plant life. Building sites and derelict houses also harbour a wide variety of medicinal plants. Yes, there is atmospheric pollution in cities, lead and carbon monoxide to name two of the deadliest, but the countryside is equally polluted these days. Most of my friends who are country dwellers live within spillage distance of a nuclear power plant; land is often sprayed from the air by nitrates used in intensive farming techniques (which also pollute the watertable). The illusion that the countryside is cleaner than the city cannot really be sustained. We could instead buy organic plants, which are generally guaranteed to be free from pesticides and fertilizers, but these too will have absorbed atmospheric pollution. Pollution is with us; we can, however, minimize its effects.

Collecting herbs

1. Choose your plants carefully, using an illustrated herbal identification guide if necessary. Always collect from a clump of plants; this shows you that the soil conditions are right for the plant and that the pollution is not too bad.
2. Plants may be rinsed quickly after picking, but don't soak them as this will wash out the water-soluble parts of the plants.
3. A student in one of my evening classes gave me this recipe for reducing the effects of pollution: add one cup of cider vinegar to one gallon of water, then wash the plant in this solution.
4. Bear in mind that we can also be polluters. When you pick your plants, never uproot them unless you need the root. In England it is illegal to uproot any plant, although no one will mind the odd dandelion or burdock root. Be sure to leave behind enough for the next herbalist who comes along – and for next year's growth too.

PICKING THE PLANTS

Herbs are at their best just as the flower buds are beginning to open. The time depends on the individual plant, but it is usually from May to September. Roots are dug either in November or December when the sap has been drawn down, or March, before it rises again. Berries and seeds are collected in their own season, when they are at their most potent.

Don't collect plants in plastic bags, as the plant material will react with the chemicals in the plastic and plant material ferments really quickly in the heat of plastic. Use wicker baskets or paper bags.

When collecting roots, be sure to cut them up before drying as they can become very hard when dry, making cutting very difficult.

DRYING YOUR PLANTS

Herbs are best dried out of direct sunlight, in a warm, dry, well-ventilated place. Airing cupboards and garden sheds are ideal. They need plenty of circulating air to dry thoroughly and to prevent mildew. Tie them in small bunches and hang them from coat hangers. Be sure to label everything, because once dried, plants can be difficult to tell apart. Depending on the weather (or rather the humidity), plants will take between 6-8 weeks to dry. Test them by breaking a stem. If it makes a clean break, they are dry; if not, you need to wait. Roots can be dried spread out on newspaper, as can seeds and berries. As pleasant as they may look, don't hang herbs in your kitchen to dry. Cooking smells and fats will stick to them, making them useless as medicine.

STORAGE

Store herbs away from direct sunlight and in a damp-free place – not the refrigerator. Put them either in dark glass jars, paper bags or wooden containers. Again, don't use plastic containers, as herbs contain volatile oils that react with plastic.

Dried herbs usually last from one season to the next, that is a year. Sometimes they will last longer. The best way to tell is to smell and taste the plant. The aromatic plants, such as lavender and rosemary, should have their characteristic smell, as should the bitters. If the plant has lost its colour or taste, it is no longer useful for medicinal purposes. Be sure to label and date your herbs.

HERBAL PREPARATIONS

There are almost as many ways to prepare herbal remedies as there are ways to bake a cake, and the comparison is far from coincidental. Making medicines has much in common with cooking and should be approached in the same spirit – one of experimentation and fun. The dose ranges that I recommend come from my personal experience of working with plants: again, different herbalists use different quantities. One thing I have learned through experience is that low doses often work better than high doses, that more does not necessarily mean better. However, it is hard to overdose with herbs. As long as you follow my guidelines and are sure of your identifications you will be safe. Obviously, one has to use one's common sense, but sticking to the common herbs, especially if you have picked them yourself, has no risk. One of the problems has been that unscrupulous suppliers have mixed different species together; for example, several years back one sample of comfrey, was found to contain aconite (which is very poisonous) when examined. This is another good reason to make your own medicines.

HERBAL TEAS

For me, this is the best way to take herbal remedies, especially if you have access to the fresh plant.

½ oz (12.5g) dried herb/root, or a handful of the freshly-chopped plant
1 pint (500ml) boiling water

Mix the two and cover and leave to brew for at least 10 minutes. Sip the mixture throughout the day.

You may sweeten herbal teas with a touch of honey, unless they are bitter teas (used for the liver or stomach), in which case take them unsweetened.

If you need an extra strong brew, for an emergency or a really serious condition, mix the herb with cold water, bring it to the boil, cover the pan and simmer for 10 minutes. Most herbs are taken before meals, that is 10-15 minutes before eating.

It is best to use a heat-resistant glass, ceramic or non-stick saucepan for preparing herbs, rather than a metal pan, as the herbs may react with the metal, especially aluminium.

TINCTURES

These are concentrated herbal essences. They are stronger, last longer and are easier to take. They are particularly useful for children who often won't drink herb teas, babies and the very ill. Traditionally, tinctures are made with ethyl alcohol, but medicinal alcohol or a spirit-based drink such as gin or vodka will do just as well. I use glycerol (glycerine) for my tinctures, as it has a pleasant taste and has no harmful effects on alcohol-sensitive people. Whichever you choose, the proportions and method remain the same. (Vegetable glycerol is available through medical suppliers but is very expensive.)

1 oz (25g) dried herb
5 fl oz (150ml) boiling water
½ pt (250ml) alcohol or glycerol

Mix all the ingredients in a large glass jar. Push the contents well down so the liquid covers the herbs (or else they will go mouldy). Label the container and put it aside for a month. From time to time during that month, shake the contents to mix everything evenly, always making sure that the herbs are covered by the liquid. When the month is up, strain out the liquid and discard the herb. If you plan to make a lot of tinctures, you would be advised to invest in a wine press to make extraction easier. Bottle in dark glass jars and label. Store away from the heat and sunlight.

Dose: adults: 5-10 drops three times daily before meals; children: 1-5 drops three times daily; babies: 1-2 drops in milk or juice three times daily. For acute conditions and in emergencies, up to 15 drops eight times daily for not more than three days.

EXTERNAL REMEDIES

HERBAL OILS

Plants extract well in oils, which can then be used as a base for ointments or on their own.

The basic method is as follows:

1 pint (500ml) oil (I use extra virgin olive oil, but almond, sunflower or unperfumed massage oil will do)
1 oz (25g) dried herb

Mix the ingredients together in a wide-mouthed glass jar, then stand in direct sunlight, for 4-6 weeks. The sunlight will extract the active principles of the plant and dissolve them into the oil.

When there is no sunlight, or you need the oil quickly, follow the following method: stand the jar (with the same ingredients) in a double boiler or bain-marie for 4-6 hours. The heat will extract the active principles.

In either case, after the extraction process has finished, strain the liquid and bottle.

This oil can be used on its own as a massage oil or made into a cream.

CREAMS

1 pint (500ml) infused oil (see above recipe)
3-4 tablespoons lanolin or cocoa butter
2 oz (50g) beeswax

Warm the oil slightly and melt in the lanolin or cocoa butter and beeswax. Remove from heat and beating well, allow the mixture to cool and thicken into a cream. To make the cream stronger, you can add ¼-½ fl oz (10-20ml) of tincture. These creams are on the oily side but work very well.

LOTIONS

Use a lotion where the skin is hot and itchy and needs to be cooled down – for example, rashes, inflammationss or skin irritations. Any of the flower waters will do, although their properties vary: rose water and orange flower water are soothing and healing, as is chamomile water. Witch-hazel is more astringent and drying. These flower waters are excellent for the mucous membranes, the mouth, throat and vagina. Any combination of tinctures can be mixed with the flower water in the ratio one part tincture to ten parts water. They will keep almost indefinitely, but I generally make them up as required.

Enjoy being creative with your herbs, invent and enjoy!

2 Puberty

PUBERTY IS THE first stage of womanhood. Although many girls feel and to all purposes remain children when they begin to menstruate, the first period signals the ending of childhood and the possibility of pregnancy and motherhood.

The age at which a girl begins to menstruate varies and is to a large part dependent upon her body weight. The first bleed shows that the girl is now able to bear a child, and to sustain pregnancy a certain amount of body fat is needed. Thus as we grow larger and our children become taller and more well-developed, puberty begins earlier and earlier.

One might suppose that today, in the late twentieth century, there are no secrets about the function of a woman's body, but sadly, this is not the case. Ignorance is still widespread and the superstitions and myths surrounding menstruation remain as powerful as always.

There are orthodox groups within the major religions which have very strict taboos surrounding menstrual blood. Women at their periods are considered to be unclean, the blood is seen as dirty and possessing power to harm. Contact between the sexes is proscribed, women should not prepare food, cut their hair or wash it, and have the power to turn milk and wine sour and generally wreak havoc. Many religions also insist that after their bleeding has finished, women undergo a cleansing ritual to make them 'fit' to have sexual intercourse and carry on the rest of their normal lives. In aboriginal communities, menstruating women went to a hut during this time. This practice has much to recommend it. I am sure many women would love to take themselves off for five days each month, away from the demands of family to be with themselves and their fertile bodies. However, most ordinary women are expected to continue as normal and to pretend that nothing is happening.

Whichever extreme applies to your particular life, taboo or denial, the beliefs about menstruation profoundly affect how we feel about this natural function.

My contention is that many of the common menstrual disorders have their roots in emotional and psychic beliefs. If one subscribes to the belief that menstruation is dirty, that women are unclean, toxic, capable of putrefying food, then how does one view those parts of one's body where this blood comes from? Logically, one would see oneself as dirty, polluted and in need of cleansing and view the natural process with disgust, fear and perhaps anger.

Many adolescent girls view the onset of menstruation as a 'curse', the name my mother's generation gave to periods: a bloody, messy episode to deal with each month, with tampons, pads, cramps and the risk and responsibility of fertility. Such negativity may well have an effect on the physical organs themselves, causing cramps, missed periods and discharges. An adolescent girl, really still a child, enters into this minefield quite ignorant of the force of feeling which surrounds her natural biological functions. She will, in whatever society or culture she belongs to, have grown up with shame about her body and yet at the same time, awe at its power to drive men crazy and cause them to do the most irrational and bizarre things. Her body is both a precious prize to be protected at all costs and at the same time, dirty, ridiculous and second rate. It is no wonder, then, that these extreme double messages rebound onto her physical being, acting out the conflict at another level.

I remember, when I began to menstruate, watching my mother burn the bloody pads and wondering just how such a seemingly innocuous liquid could be so dangerous that it needed to be burned in a fire at the bottom of the garden. Or later, being at Guide camp and putting a used tampon in a special bin, only to be severely reprimanded for not carefully wrapping it up, lest the younger girls saw it. Luckily, my response was to consider all adults quite mad and to take no notice whatsoever, but many girls absorb this shame and fear, and use it to punish their bodies.

Anorexia, which is a complex emotional disorder, has its roots in the denial of womanhood. Anorexics cease to menstruate once their weight has dropped below a certain level. By sheer force of will, the anorexic is able to stop the maturation process and curtail her bleeding. She is able to control nature and gain a sense of power over her seemingly out-of-control body. But of course, the price to pay is high; anorexics centre their lives around this obsession with food, may end up in psychiatric units or even die of the disease.

Of course, the majority of girls don't have such extreme reactions, but internally, the conflict continues and the body is often the battlefield. For this reason, it is vital that we educate young girls and give them a positive image of themselves as women and their reproductive functions. We need to counter the propaganda, prejudices and ignorance surrounding menstruation, and like our matriarchal foremothers, recognize it as a sacred time, a quiet time and a purifying time.

It would be useful here to look at some of the physical aspects of menstruation. What is it, and where does the blood come from?

Menstruation comes about as the lining of the womb (endometrium) is shed. This lining is rich with blood vessels which will sustain and nourish a child, should one be conceived. When conception does not occur, the lining and tiny blood vessels separate from the walls of the uterus and pass out of the body. This is the menstrual blood which, clearly, is no dirtier than any other blood, although it is true to say that the colour and consistency of the blood does change from month to month and according to one's state of health. Therefore from the colour, consistency and quantity of the blood loss, one can tell a good deal about a woman's state of health.

COLOUR

The blood should be bright red in colour, like the blood which comes from a cut blood vessel. This shows that there is a good oxygen supply to the uterus and that the circulation is functioning well. Very light, pinkish-red blood might mean anaemia, low blood pressure or poor circulation. Dark red or brown blood generally signifies poor circulation and pelvic congestion; the larger the blood clots, the worse the congestion. Clots can also signify a discharge around the cervix, which catches the blood as it drips from the womb, causing it to coagulate and clot. Meat eaters tend to have darker blood than vegetarians, so this must also be taken into consideration when examining menstrual blood.

During or after an illness the blood will be darker, as it will be if the diet is poor, consisting of large amounts of sugar, meat, chemical foods and alcohol. The colour of your blood is like a barometer, indicating the state of your reproductive system, circulation and also the organs of elimination, the liver and kidneys.

QUANTITY

This again is an indication of the general state of health of a woman. The average period lasts 5 days and is heaviest on the first day (sometimes the second), gradually tailing off by the 5th day. If a woman needs to change her tampon or pad more than every 2-3 hours, the flow can be considered to be heavy. In the same way, the blood loss is seen as slight if there is no need, other than out of preference, to change more than twice daily. Women generally know what is normal for them, and that really is the best guide. Girls at puberty have no such guide, but mostly we follow the same pattern as our mothers.

Heavy bleeding (menorrhagia) is common at puberty, but need not be endured. It can be regulated by herbal remedies, for if it is allowed to continue, it will cause anaemia and low blood pressure, to which adolescent girls are prone (see the section on Heavy bleeding and Anaemia, pages 53-55).

Too light a flow, while not harmful, is nevertheless an indication that all is not as it should be. Perhaps there is anaemia, low blood pressure or general weakness and debility. In either case, a course of treatment with a herbal tonic will right the imbalance.

IRREGULAR CYCLES

This is a common complaint. Some girls have cycles of three weeks, then seven, then five. The problem is similar to that encountered in the menopause, except here the hormonal cycle is beginning and finding its feet, and really these are minor hiccoughs. As the liver adjusts itself to breaking down these hormones each month, the cycle should regulate itself (see the section on PMT (pages 44-49 for an explanation of the liver's role in hormone levels). If the problem persists, a herbal hormonal remedy which also acts on the liver is recommended; marigold is the remedy of choice, but also helpful are: mugwort, sage, lady's mantle, false unicorn root, wild yam and squaw vine. To regulate the cycle, the remedy has to be taken for at least three months before any real change will be seen.

PAINFUL PERIODS

Again a common problem, in part caused by anxiety, leading to tension in the uterus. Usually the pain is spasmodic and needs relaxant remedies to ease it. Exercise is important, especially the yoga postures for opening the pelvis: see page 85-86. Remedies particularly helpful for girls at puberty include: mugwort, yarrow, archangel, cramp bark, blue cohosh, raspberry leaf, and skullcap (see the section on Painful periods on page 49).

DISCHARGES

Often girls at puberty have a discharge which is non-specific and is known as leucorrhoea. It is unclear why certain women have more of a discharge than others. Diet, temperament, hormones and the general level of health all play an important part in causing discharges. A diet high in dairy produce, sugar, refined carbohydrates and animal fats produces mucus, resulting in a predisposition to discharges. A small amount of discharge is normal, particularly in the middle of the menstrual cycle and premenstrually. A healthy discharge is normally white or colourless, and odourless. Yellowish, greenish or blood-stained discharges are definitely abnormal and need to be investigated. Cheesy-smelling discharges suggest thrush; those with a putrid smell usually indicate an infection of some kind (see Thrush, page 61, and Trichamoniasis, page 62).

SKIN CHANGES

Hormones also affect the skin, although their role is perhaps a little overplayed. Hormonal changes are a cause of acne, but not the main one. Diet is very important here, animal fats, dairy produce, sugar and alcohol all cause bad skin and need to be eliminated or reduced to a minimum. Conversely, fresh fruit and vegetables clear the skin, as does drinking a lot of pure (spring/filtered) water; ten glasses daily with a little lemon juice is recommended. Exercise increases the blood flow to the skin, bringing oxygen and nutrients and taking away waste products, and thus has a cleansing function. A useful remedy for both the skin and the hormonal system is marigold; for mild skin problems, archangel, echinacea and gentian root are helpful; if the problem is severe, use vitex with a liver remedy such as dandelion root.

CONCLUSION

Puberty is a shock to the system and affects the body in the same way as pregnancy and the menopause. It takes time for the body to adjust to the new rhythm and to acclimatize itself to losing blood each month. The rise and fall of hormone levels affect not only the physical body, but the emotions as well. This is a time fraught with challenges as a young girl's body begins to change from girl into woman, and her status in society changes accordingly. Treatment should be a combination of gentle herbal remedies to redress any hormonal imbalance, a healthy lifestyle and positive psychological input to counter society's misogynist view of women. The experience of an older woman is vital at this stage. Girls need to have women talk to them about the positive aspects of being a woman to strengthen their self-image, boost their self-esteem and create a new generation of bold, beautiful women.

3   The Menopause

THE MENOPAUSE, OR climacteric, is the medical terminology for the years in which a woman's body is adjusting to declining hormone levels. Naturally, this changes the body, but these changes have been exaggerated and distorted by both the medical profession and everyday prejudices.

The change of life comes at a critical time in the lives of most women. From 45-55, most women who have been biological mothers gradually see their work reduce as their offspring leave home or grow up enough to need little of the intensive care and attention that they did previously. If a woman has not become a biological mother, the menopause marks the final point beyond which biological motherhood ceases to be possible. For a woman with a career, these years often represent the culmination of their work, and the rewards (or otherwise) that it brings. Clearly, then, this time brings up issues surrounding women's identity, their role in society and the success they feel they have achieved in the world.

At the same time, the ageing process becomes more visible. Lines, wrinkles and loose muscles become more evident and less easy to cover up. If a woman has lived very much from the power her physical appearance has given her, this time will represent a real watershed in her life. Perhaps because of the way our society views old age, many women dread ageing, and the powerlessness they see accompanying it. Women often fight back against ageing with harsh exercise regimes, starving themselves anorexically thin and taking artificial hormones to keep younger. Their denial of their ageing process is seen as a normal, correct response.

On the other hand, women who refuse to deny their ageing process often find that they become invisible almost overnight. Older friends of mine have noticed that younger women and men attract more attention than themselves, but they are not supposed to complain; if they do complain, they are labelled as crazy old women and are simply seen as fulfilling a stereotype.

In neither case are women given the respect older women find in other cultures. In the West older people, and women in particular, are seen as 'past it', useless, good for nothing. The wisdom that has come through living out their lives is not respected. Because we are cut off from our roots and our instincts, we do not value the living past; older people, as representatives of that past, are feared and despised, perhaps because they remind us that there is nothing new under the sun.

Women, besides suffering discrimination through ageing, also suffer discrimination for being women. Thus an older woman, who can no longer be idealized as a beauty, or admired as a young mother, often has her status reduced in advertising and the media to that of granny, another gross stereotype. The image of a strong older woman existing in her own right is rarely portrayed on television, film or in literature. The question facing us is how much of what is labelled 'the menopause' relates to the physical manifestations, and how much is a result of the ageing process.

WHAT IS THE MENOPAUSE?

Clinically, this is said to be when a woman's hormone levels decrease, her periods become increasingly irregular and finally cease altogether. The medical definition of the menopause is said to be 6-9 months after the periods have stopped. The age of the climacteric varies; it is usually from 45-55, although it is getting later. There are a whole variety of symptoms associated with the menopause, or believed to be connected to this fall-off in hormone levels; I say this because there is doubt as to which symptoms can be abscribed to hormone levels and which are stress-related. One physician has declared that there is no such thing as the menopause. However, I have listed below the commonest complaints associated with the change of life which remain real problems, whether we would call them menopausal or not.

HEAVY BLEEDING

Generally, this is the first sign that the menopause is approaching. The cycles change in length, becoming further apart, or closer together. Sometimes the periods become lighter and tail off, other times they become heavier. Heavy bleeding is often seen as a sign that a hysterectomy is needed. Although it is true to say that heavy and prolonged periods will cause inconvenience to a woman's life, hysterectomy is a serious operation and should only be undertaken as a last resort. Heavy periods can be a sign of other illnesses, notably fibroids and endometriosis. It is less often a sign of cancer. The main problem caused by heavy bleeding is anaemia (see Heavy bleeding & Anaemia, pages 53-55).

HOT FLUSHES

Much talked about and often dreaded, hot flushes give a sensation of heat in the face which is often accompanied by profuse sweating. There may be a feeling of suffocation, followed by chills.

The woman experiencing the hot flush often feels highly self-conscious but generally other people don't notice anything, other than a slight heightening of colour. Much of the embarrassment is due to their sudden and unpredictable nature.

Flushes are aggravated by cigarettes, sugar, tea, coffee, alcohol and spices.

TREATMENT

When you feel a flush coming on, for example if you are rushing for a deadline or in a hot crowded atmosphere, try not to fight it, but relax into it – the less tense you are, the less severe the flush will be. As the hands and wrists heat and cool the body rapidly, run cold water over the wrists to cool down. Try to wear several layers of light cotton clothing.

The lists of suggested herbal treatments below are classified as 'mild' or 'severe', depending on the type of condition.

Mild:

St John's wort, melissa, sage.

Severe:

Vitex, lavender, marigold, hawthorn.

EMOTIONAL CHANGES

As outlined above, it is hard to know which symptoms can be ascribed to the menopause and which would appear as a reaction to the ageing process. Women are often said to become depressed during the menopause, and somehow I feel there is an implicit message that this is quite likely to happen, given the nature of the situation, the stresses that a menopausal woman is under and the way in which society at large responds to psychological distress. It is to be expected that her emotional distress is put down to having physical causes, which is easier to accept and less likely to rock the boat. We could therefore suspect that depression, anxiety and anger might be different reactions to the same stresses. Statistics show that poor women, black women and immigrant women are far more likely to be diagnosed as depressed than wealthy white women, thus it could be argued that depression is more of a socio-economic disease than an emotional one. The same statistics apply to anxiety; tranquillizer prescriptions tend to go to the poorest women and especially to women over 45.

Having said all this, it is true that physical therapy can help psychological conditions. Diet plays a vital role in one's emotional well-being. Excess sugar in the diet, stimulants, alcohol and drugs will all contribute to a deteriorating psychological state (see Hypoglycaemia, page 47, for a discussion of sugar and depression). Coffee, tea and caffeine drinks all aggravate anxiety: taken in excess, they will cause lethargy and irritability. Alcohol is a well-known depressant and should be avoided. Eat as well as you are able. Try to get as much protein as you can; a wholefood diet and additive-free regime will also reduce irritation to the nervous tissue. Exercise is invaluable in treating both depression and anxiety, although it is probably the last thing you feel like doing. Actually making the effort to do something physical is both relaxing and invigorating: it calms the mind, lifts the spirits and need not be hard work or boring. Dancing, walking and running are all cheap forms of pleasurable, if not entirely painless exercise.

REMEDIES

Depression

Mild: melissa, yarrow, motherwort
Severe: vitex, rosemary, ginger

Anxiety

Mild: melissa, motherwort
Severe: lavender, hypericum, lime flowers, skullcap

IMPORTANT

Any woman who has been taking any prescription drugs for depression or anxiety (antidepressants or tranquillizers) must not suddenly stop the drugs and replace them with herbal remedies. Sudden withdrawal of these drugs can cause a crisis - the symptoms for which the drug was originally prescribed may well return but with much more severity. If you want to stop taking tranquillizers and change to herbal remedies, slowly reduce the dose over a period of several weeks at the same time as taking the herbal remedy. The two will not interact and can safely be taken side by side.

INSOMNIA

This is often a by-product of depression and anxiety, although it can appear independently of either. Nightsweats and palpitations will increase the likelihood of insomnia. Insomnia should be treated in the same way as anxiety by cutting down on stimulants and increasing exercise. Herbal remedies should be taken half an hour before retiring.

TREATMENT

Mild

Melissa, motherwort

Severe

Lavender, lime flowers, skullcap

HORMONE REPLACEMENT

The medical profession tends to respond to the menopause as it does to pregnancy and childbirth, often taking drastic and interventionist action as a preventative measure. Hysterectomy, HRT, tranquillizers and antidepressants are all routinely prescribed to the menopausal woman. Often these remedies are more dangerous and their side-effects more damaging than the conditions they are supposed to treat.

Hormone treatments have been used for forty years on menopausal women. There has been an aggressive campaign to promote and sell these drugs, to the extent that in the USA, premarin (for HRT) has become the fifth most prescribed wonder remedy. HRT was hailed as another wonder drug, stopping hot flushes, vaginal dryness, heart disease and cancer. It was also claimed to reverse the ageing process, increase libido and stop osteoporosis. Needless to say, inadequate medical trials failed to highlight the dangers of long-term use. These risks have proved to be similar to those found with the contraceptive pill: a woman using HRT has a 5-15 times higher risk of endometrial cancer, especially if she has been on the drug for more than a year. It has also been found that claims originally made for HRT have not been substantiated and the only demonstrable effects have been against flushes and vaginal dryness, both of which are directly related to low oestrogen levels.

As with the pill, women with certain diseases should not take HRT; neither should women who have a history of breast disease, cancer, blood clots, arteriosclerosis, heart, liver or kidney disease and who smoke. It has been estimated that women using HRT for 7-10 years double the risk of developing breast cancer. HRT also increases the risk of developing fibroids. Some women have reported that HRT helped their symptoms when used for a short time. Others said that after stopping the drug, their symptoms returned, and were worse than ever.

THE HERBAL APPROACH

The menopause is not seen as a disease, but simply a change in conditions and another stage in a woman's life. As such, it needs the minimum of intervention. Short-term treatment, together with simple dietary advice and a sane psychological approach, is what is needed.

HERBAL HORMONES

There are several herbal remedies which contain substances which act on the body in the same way as hormones. They occur naturally in plants and tend to adapt themselves to imbalances in the body – if, for example, there is a lack of oestrogen, they have an oestrogenic action. Others are more specific; one herb, vitex, acts like progesterone. Below is a list of the more easily-available herbal hormone remedies.

Oestrogens

False unicorn root, red clover, black and blue cohosh, marigold, sage, wild yam, liquorice root

Progesterone

Vitex

Androgens

Sarsaparilla, damiana

Generally speaking, during the menopause women need oestrogen to help the body adapt to the lowered levels in the body. Herbal hormonal remedies are safer because they are balanced out by other substances in the plant. They are not as strong as synthetic hormones, nor are they hormones in isolation. Plants are powerfully-acting pharmacological agents, but they work slowly. Generally, any remedy has to be used for at least three months to see an effect, but once they act, their effects are long-lasting. Herbs are not used as substitutes for drugs, nor are they intended to be used indefinitely. The aim is to rebalance the system and slowly reduce the dosage until the body functions as it should without the remedy.

This is important, as women on HRT are expected to take it for the rest of their lives. This, together with the fact that 70 per cent of prescription drugs are prescribed to women over 45, indicates the current medical approach to the menopause. I have treated many women complaining of menopausal symptoms, from severe to mild. The great majority cleared up within three to six months on low doses of tinctures.

OTHER COMMON MENOPAUSAL AILMENTS

VAGINAL DRYNESS

This is due to a combination of factors, including the fall in oestrogen levels and the effect of ageing on the mucous membranes. Treatment for this is hormonally based. I have found a mixture of marigold and lady's mantle very helpful, together with a light cream or lotion of marigold applied internally. Motherwort and mugwort may be added to the mixture as general gynaecological tonics.

DRY SKIN

Again, this is due both to hormones and to the ageing process. An internal mixture of marigold, red clover and melissa is useful. Take care to use only natural cosmetics on the skin. Calendula cream may be used externally to soften the skin.

BRITTLE BONE SYNDROME

This is the thinning of the bones, a process which begins in the twenties but gets worse as the hormone levels drop. Diet and exercise particularly anti-gravity exercise – e.g. swimming – play an important role in its treatment and prevention. A lifetime of rigorous dieting may well seriously deplete the body of basic vitamins and minerals, and when the menopause comes on top of this it precipitates a crisis. There are several herbal remedies which increase the mineral content of the blood and help to build bone tissue: horsetail for silica, nettles for iron & vitamin C, comfrey for vitamin B12 and allantoin.

Always take with one of the bitter remedies – dandelion, marigold or yarrow – to increase absorption.

CIRCULATORY PROBLEMS

Our hormones also affect the circulation of the blood and women tend to suffer from a variety of circulatory changes as they grow older. Oestrogen is again implicated here. Hypertension (see High blood pressure, page 56) and varicose veins are the most common. The treatment approach is twofold: first use a hormonal balancer such as marigold, lady's mantle or vitex and then add a remedy for the heart and circulation such as yarrow or hawthorn for hypertension and circulatory problems and melissa or motherwort for palpitations. If you feel the palpitations are stress-related, add relaxants like melissa, lime flowers or yarrow.

PROLAPSE

This is the collapse or semi-collapse of the vaginal wall, allowing the vagina to slip down. It causes a dragging feeling and may cause cystitis, incontinence, pain and heavy bleeding. The best treatment is pelvic floor exercises (see Exercises, page 85) combined with herbal astringents such as shepherd's purse and hypericum. A douche of sage tea once daily is useful.

LOSS OF LIBIDO

Some women do complain of a lessening interest in sex at the menopause. There is no particular reason why this should be so, although some writers again claim oestrogen as the culprit. Sexuality is a subject large enough for a book on its own, if not several, and so complex that a purely physical treatment is unlikely to provide the answer. Both marigold and lady's mantle have a reputation for increasing the libido and may be worth a try. Vitex, on the other hand, is said to decrease the libido.

DIET DURING THE MENOPAUSE

As for all the other stages of life, a healthy sensible diet is essential and will do much to alleviate both physical and emotional symptoms. Ageing changes our bodily needs and also the ways in which we digest and use the foods we eat.

1. *Metabolic rate.* The older we get, the fewer calories we need. This is because our metabolic rate slows down and we generally take less exercise and do less physical work.
2. *Weight gain.* Because of the above, women tend to gain weight – on average 10 lbs (4.5kg). This is not due to the menopause itself, but presumably to changes in lifestyle. There are advantages and disadvantages in this weight gain: the thinner a woman is, the more likely she is to get osteoporosis, as fat tissue has been found to contain androgens which are converted to oestrogens after the menopause. On the other hand, overweight women are more likely to suffer from diabetes and high blood pressure, as well as problems with their weight-bearing joints. Ignore the weight charts and decide for yourself if you need to lose weight.

Questions to ask yourself include whether you feel healthy and fit; whether your energy levels altered recently; and whether you have normal blood pressure, blood sugar, and blood cholesterol. Your answers will tell you more about your general level of health than any chart.

3. *Absorption.* As the body ages, it is less able to absorb and digest food. This means that potential vitamins and minerals are lost. Supplements can be taken but it is better still to have a regular routine of taking a bitter tonic to stimulate digestion and the absorption of foods. This can be taken as a herbal tea, or as a tincture. Commonly available bitter tinctures include chamomile, dandelion root and melissa. Bitters must taste bitter to work, so don't sweeten them with honey. Take the tincture or tea 20-30 minutes before meals.

4. *Protein.* We need more protein as we get older, as our tissues need replacing at a greater rate. Increase your protein intake, and if you are a vegetarian, be sure to check you are combining your foods properly (see the section on Diet, pages 79-84).

5. *Calcium.* This prevents bone loss, a great risk for the menopausal woman. It is harder for women over 35 to absorb calcium. Exercise helps absorption, together with a diet high in calcium and low in phosphorus, which causes a loss of calcium from the bones; it is found in meat and cola drinks. Magnesium is needed to absorb calcium, and we also need more of this as we age; 1500mg of calcium, 750mg of magnesium and 400 IU of vitamin D are needed daily. See the vitamin chart on page 86.

6. *Constipation.* This can be a problem during this time: fibre and increased exercise levels help, as does increasing fluid levels to at least six glasses of water daily.

7. *Fat.* As we grow older, the risks from eating fat increase and at the same time, the long-term effects of meat eating begin to take their toll. Have your cholesterol levels checked

regularly and if they are raised, cut down on all animal fats, dairy produce, nuts and eggs and take more exercise. Certain herbal remedies have been found to help lower cholesterol levels, including garlic, lime flowers and yarrow.

EXERCISE

Exercise becomes very important, especially as we grow older. It increases calcium absorption, strengthens the bones, muscles and tissues of the body. It has a tranquillizing effect on the body and helps reduce anxiety and insomnia. It lowers blood pressure, reduces arteriosclerosis and reduces the risk of a heart attack. The best way of slowing the ageing process is to make sure you have a healthy diet and plenty of exercise.

CONCLUSION

I hope I have shown in this chapter that the menopause is not simply a slow decline towards death, and that it is best approached in a positive and creative spirit.

The image we have of the older woman is at great variance with how they are seen in more traditional societies. In these societies, women have a clearer role as they grow old; they are freer and less subject to taboos than women who are still menstruating. Because of this, they are strong, wise in their own way and command great respect within the community. Here in the West we need to re-create the image of the powerful matriarch who may or may not be the head of a family. For ourselves and our daughters, it is vital that this change of life heralds a wise age in the life of women, and is neither denied by pill or surgery, nor collapsed into as being one step from the grave.

4 Common Gynaecological Problems

THE ILLNESSES I have included in this chapter are those which I have come across most frequently in my clinical practice. They cover most of the field of gynaecology, although other systems are involved too.

The chapter on puberty (page 22) describes how menstrual blood is a good indicator of the general level of health of an individual. Go back to that section for a description of different types of menstrual flow.

Besides the loss of blood, how a period manifests itself also indicates the general health level of a woman. Associated with the period are five main conditions: premenstrual tension (PMT), painful periods, heavy periods, irregular periods and the absence of periods.

PRE-MENSTRUAL TENSION

The symptoms of PMT vary from woman to woman. PMT tends to become more severe after the age of 25; the reasons for this are unclear, but include greater emotional sensitivity, less stable hormone levels and a generally lower standard of health and of the liver in particular.

Symptoms occur 7-10 days before the period begins and increase in severity until bleeding starts. They include one or more of the following: bloating and water retention, tiredness, insomnia, irritability, depression, a hunger for sugar and carbohydrates, headache, migraine, acne and pimples.

Pre-menstrual women are more emotionally vulnerable and very sensitive. Women who are creative – artists, writers and musicians – report that pre-menstrually they experience an upsurge in ideas. They dream more, have more creative insights and are more easily in touch with their particular muse. Other women (sadly, the majority) suffer from irritability and emotional outbursts. I think the above gives us a clue about the genesis and possible treatment strategies, but we have to go a little deeper into the issue before we can look at ways in which to approach the illness.

As women, we are cyclical beings. Our menstrual rhythms change us physically, emotionally and mentally in the space of one short month. This has made us more adaptable, more fluid and less rigid. Before we lived in an industrialized world, women were able to alter their rhythms to rural life – the pace was slower, there was more flexibility and one could describe the physical world as being more in tune with female energies. As society became industrialized and we began to work to a clock, to a working week, in offices, shops, factories and schools, we needed to squash the broadness of our experience into a smaller slot. Now we all have to work to time, to schedules, to long-range plans. We exist in a linear world, where time marches in straight lines and the cyclical rhythmic reality of the lunar, and indeed, menstrual, existence has no place.

If it is true that when we are pre-menstrual we are more creative and more receptive to our femininity, it is not at all surprising that we crash headlong into this linear, regimented ordered world. We have to fight to survive, and, because as women we still lack the strength to fight on our own terms, we end up fighting ourselves and our bodies, exhorting them to behave themselves.

As we rush through supermarket queues and rush hour traffic, as we try to pack into our lives all that is needed to survive in our world, our instincts tell us to rest, to dream and to be creative. And because of the way modern life is organized, or more rightly, because life is not organized in our favour, tension is created.

We are more likely than men to burst into tears with frustration as we miss the bus, get jostled in the street, or react with rage to the 'normal' aggressive behaviour to which women are subjected. One could argue that our reactions are sane and that the world is mad. But most women have to live in this man-made real world, and to run home and family and work generally unaided. Life outside is dangerous for women (one only has to look at rape statistics). Pollutants such as noise, hurry and aggression wear us down daily and we have precious little time to call our own, let alone space to develop and grow. That is, socio-economic factors are vitally important. If PMT manifests itself as frustration, logically one should look for causes of that frustration in the life of the women complaining of it. And easy it would be to find.

But, I hear you asking, how is this going to help me through next month's ordeal of swollen breasts, heaviness, tiredness and bad temper? Well, in one way, it can't, unless we start a revolution today and change the world. In another way, it can. Understanding, I always feel, is half-way to solving a problem. If you can, next month, remember that it is the world that is mad, and not you, it might just help to put your experiences into perspective.

But the physical is important, too: our physical bodies affect our feelings, and vice versa. If we are healthy physically, chances are that our emotions will be more stable and less likely to be running riot.

THE ROLE OF THE LIVER

Physically PMT is caused by high levels of hormones circulating in the blood stream. At ovulation (approximately day 14 of the menstrual cycle) these hormone levels peak and thereafter they usually reduce quite suddenly. In PMT, for various reasons, this reduction of hormone levels does not occur and higher levels than normal are found in the blood. Generally, it is oestrogen which is the culprit, and conventional treatment is aimed at countering this by giving the hormone progesterone.

This could be described as using a sledge-hammer to crack a nut, and my instinct has always been one of great caution in the use of any synthetic hormone. The hormone levels in our bodies are miniscule but likewise, tiny amounts can affect us tremendously. We must, then, ask the question why these hormone levels are raised.

In my opinion, the fault is not often to do with the secretion of hormones, but with the liver, the mechanism which is supposed to break them down. For it is the liver's role in the body to break down and pass out toxic and unwanted substances. Everything we take into our bodies, including substances in the air we breathe, at some stage passes through the liver. It is like a huge processing plant, sorting out the good from the bad, and helpful from the harmful and sending the end products to other parts of the body for storage, use or excretion.

Given the environment we now live in – our toxic and polluted planet, the drugs we use, from caffeine and nicotine to the pharmaceuticals we are prescribed, the adulterated and genetically engineered food we eat, with its preservatives, colourants, additives and detoxicants – you can imagine how worn out, if not plain exhausted, our livers must be.

I always treat the livers of all patients who come to me, because however pure their diet, they live with atmospheric pollutants and their livers will probably be stressed.

Treatment is one end of the story and prevention the other. It figures that if women reduce their intake of poisons, the strain on their liver will be reduced and they will better be able to respond to the monthly shift in hormone levels.

Cut down on alcohol, cigarettes, foods with chemicals or additives; drink organic wines and eat wholefoods. Reducing both sugar and salt will stop water retention and bloating. Sugar is important here: it has no nutritional content, but actually leaches vitamins and minerals out of the body. Women often crave sugar pre-menstrually, as it gives them a short burst of energy, but later makes them more tired and irritable (see Low blood sugar, page 57).

Some sources say that women should cut down on their fluid intake to reduce water retention, but I feel the opposite is the correct course of action. The more fluid you take in, the better your kidneys work. So drink at least six glasses of water or unsweetened fruit juice daily.

To summarize: cut down on vices: alcohol, tobacco, sugar, junk food, coffee, salt and meat, and increase your intake of whole grains, fruit, vegetables and fluids.

TREATMENT

Liver remedies

Marigold, dandelion, gentian root

Hormone balancers and gynaecological tonics

Vitex, lady's mantle, marigold, false unicorn root, skullcap (the latter two are relaxants)

Herbs should be taken throughout the menstrual cycle for at least two cycles for a clear effect to be seen. For mild PMT, use a mixture of marigold and lady's mantle; for severe or long-standing PMT, use chaste berry and dandelion root, or gentian root and false unicorn root.

Herbal hormones

These are called hormones for the sake of brevity and simplicity, but they don't act like synthetic hormones and cannot be compared with them. They are more like old-fashioned tonics in that they regulate and rebalance the body, so that if there is an imbalance, they will gently right it. They take time to work, but their effects are long-lasting.

PAINFUL PERIODS (dismenorrhoea)

Is it normal to have painful periods? That I don't know, but most months, most women experience some pain. A slight dragging sensation, feeling a little weak at the knees together with odd cramps and twinges could be considered acceptable. Severe pain needing painkillers, and other symptoms such as fainting, vomiting or diarrhoea, I would consider to be abnormal. Stress, other illnesses, tiredness, poor general health and excessive use of stimulants all aggravate the pain. Conversely, relaxation techniques, tummy massage, physical exercise and orgasms reduce it.

I feel there is a strong psychogenic (emotional) component to menstrual pain. Yes, physical factors are important, but how we feel about menstruation naturally affects how it occurs. With this aim in mind I have included a simple visualization that can be done each month when bleeding begins as a way of making a positive and healthy connection with your menstrual cycle.

As the bleeding begins, or as soon as possible afterwards, take yourself off to a place where you can be undisturbed for 15-20 minutes.

Sit comfortably on the floor or on a chair. Breathe deeply and relax your whole body. On each inhalation feel yourself sinking down into your body, letting go of tension, breathing away stiff muscles. When you feel relaxed, allow your mind to centre itself on your womb. Lightly focus your attention there. Breathing deeply, let your awareness of your womb sink in deeper and deeper. Feel yourself enveloped by your muscles as you get to the centre of your womb. When you arrive, have a look around and see what is there. You may be quite surprised about what you have been storing in there. Take time to explore, check out the general condition of things and notice anything which you feel is out of place. If an image or symbol appears to you, take time to explore it; talk to it and find out what it is doing there, and why. If you have pain, imagine your womb opening out and allowing the blood to flow freely, without any obstruction. When you feel ready, bring your consciousness back into the room.

If you have serious or long-standing menstrual problems, it would be a good idea to do this exercise for several months, and to record what happens each month. This way, you will be able to see your progress and become aware of particular issues which arise for you around your womb and subject of menstruation.

Painful periods can be divided into two types, spasmodic and congestive.

SPASMODIC PERIODS

There is increased tension in the uterus and generally elsewhere in the body. The pain is sharp and intense and nausea, vomiting and diarrhoea may be accompanying symptoms. There is usually a heavy blood flow and the blood is bright red in colour.

CONGESTIVE PERIODS

Here, the pain is duller and more prolonged. The blood flow is generally heavy and dark in colour. The pain is caused by the uterus swelling with blood due to poor circulation. This pain is often relieved by heat and exercise.

Prevention

In both cases, the easiest method of prevention is exercise. Yoga (see Exercise, page 85) will stretch and relax the muscles in spasmodic dysmenorrhoea (the name for painful periods), and increase muscle tone and improve the circulation in the congestive type.

Treatment

The herbs given below can be used for symptomatic relief or for the long-term treatment of the condition.

Spasmodic: yarrow, motherwort, melissa, cramp bark, false unicorn root, squaw vine, skullcap, wild yam

Congestive: ginger, pennyroyal, false unicorn root

MISSED PERIODS (amenorrhoea)

Primary amenorrhoea is when a woman has never had a period, secondary is when for one reason or another it has not come. Primary amenorrhoea is an abnormal condition and is very difficult to treat. Secondary amenorrhoea is generally due to some trauma which temporarily shuts down the menstrual rhythm. These can include:

1. Weight loss. Women under six stone (37.5kg) do not menstruate because they do not have enough body fat to maintain a healthy pregnancy; hence this is a biological response to an abnormal situation; which is why anorexic women often have no periods.
2. Stress caused by a change of environment.

Leaving home is a classic cause of menstrual irregularities, as is becoming a student, travelling, being involved in a fight, having a serious illness, having an abortion, becoming pregnant and coming off the pill. Any kind of stress will affect the menstrual cycle. Missing the odd period or having a slightly irregular cycle is no reason to worry. When your periods fail to materialize for months on end, or where the cycle is long and completely irregular, treatment is needed.

Once pregnancy has been excluded as a cause and there has been no particular triggering factor, you should examine any possible emotional reasons for the failure to menstruate. You may have a certain amount of ambivalence, conscious or unconscious, to menstruation and to the real or imagined responsibilities that maturity brings. Pregnancy, childbirth, contraception and sexuality are all highly-charged and complex issues: it might be worth considering talking through some of your problems with a trained counsellor.

TREATMENT

Herbs cannot of course alter the external stresses, but they can reduce the effect of stress on the body.

Relaxant herbs

Mild: chamomile, melissa, motherwort
Strong: lavender, lime blossom

Gynaecological tonics

Mild: yarrow, lady's mantle, mugwort, false unicorn root, blue cohosh
Strong: vitex

Liver remedy

(after stopping the pill, or after a serious illness)
Dandelion root, marigold

HEAVY BLEEDING

This can occur at any age, but is most frequently seen at puberty and around the menopause. What constitutes heavy bleeding will depend on the norm for the individual woman. Generally, women bleed for 2-5 days, the first and second days being the heaviest. Changing pads more than hourly or during the night would indicate an excessively heavy flow, as would the presence of blood clots larger than fingernail size (see chapter 2).

Anaemia is a by-product of heavy bleeding, as is low blood-pressure.

Heavy blood loss can occur as a result of hormonal imbalance, fibroids, the menopause and puberty; most commonly, there is no known cause. I have, however, found that women who lose a lot of blood often have bad circulation and poor pelvic muscle tone. Read the section on exercises (pages 84-86) if this applies to you and follow the pelvic floor exercises.

TREATMENT

Astringents reduce blood loss and also tone up muscle tissue. Use one or more of the following as appropriate: shepherd's purse, sage, nettle.

Uterine tonics and hormonal balancers

Raspberry leaf, cramp bark, red clover, St John's wort, mugwort, lady's mantle, vitex, false unicorn root.
For the treatment of fibroids, see Serious illnesses, page 69.

ILLNESSES AFFECTING THE BLOOD AND CIRCULATION

ANAEMIA

This is where there is not enough haemoglobin in the blood to transport oxygen around the body. This cause symptoms of oxygen starvation: tiredness, dizziness, numbness in the hands and feet, shortness of breath, pallor, depression and lack of appetite. Normal levels are 12.5mm Hg in adults; levels below 10.5mm Hg are considered anaemic.

Anaemia is a symptom rather than an illness, and the most common cause is heavy blood loss in menstruation, followed by pregnancy, childbirth and breastfeeding.

Prevention

A diet rich in vitamin C and iron will prevent anaemia; the vitamin C is needed to absorb the iron. Some herbs are rich in minerals and will help to build up the blood. I once treated a woman in late pregnancy whose haemoglobin reading was an incredible 4.5mm Hg and was threatened with a blood transfusion unless she did something about it. With a mixture of melissa and nettles her haemoglobin level rose to 10.5mm Hg within ten days; no one at the hospital could believe it!

Equally, the body needs to be able to absorb the iron found in the diet, so taking a digestive stimulant will increase the amount of iron used by the body. Either dandelion or marigold will do.

Naturally, the best way of treating anaemia is to treat the underlying cause.

LOW BLOOD PRESSURE (hypotension)

Little is written about low blood pressure, partly because it is not a life-threatening condition, as is high blood pressure, and partly because there is little that can be done to break it with orthodox medicine. While it is true that low blood pressure is not a serious illness, it is nevertheless widespread among women and has a serious effect on their quality of life.

Symptoms include tiredness, irritability, exhaustion, depression, coldness, headache and low resistance to infection. Often low blood pressure co-exists with anaemia and the symptoms of both are similar. Low blood pressure does mean that the risk of heart disease is reduced; it should nevertheless be treated seriously. Normal blood pressure readings are around $\frac{110}{120}$, but I have treated women with blood pressure as low as $\frac{70}{40}$ and was amazed that they were still on their feet.

Prevention

As the medical term hypotension suggests, there is a lack of tension in the circulatory system. Stimulants are needed to increase the heart rate and speed up the circulation of the blood.

Diet can help: increase your intake of all spices, but especially ginger, the curry spices, pepper, garlic and onions as they have the effect of raising blood pressure. Exercise will increase the heart rate and make the circulation more dynamic.

Herbal circulatory stimulants raise the blood pressure and are a tonic to the circulation in general: try ginger and rosemary.

Hawthorn also raises blood pressure and increases the amount of blood the heart pumps around the body. It has a normalizing action and thus is used for both high and low blood pressure.

HIGH BLOOD PRESSURE (hypertension)

This is a far more serious condition than low blood pressure, as the possible complications – heart disease, thrombosis and stroke – are life-threatening. Hypertension used to be more prevalent among men, but it is becoming more of a problem for women. It is believed to be stress-related; anxiety pushes up the blood pressure, makes the heart beat faster and high cholesterol levels clog up the arteries, increasing the pressure in the blood vessels.

Symptoms include dizziness, ringing in the ears, fainting, headache, and pressure in the head. The majority of cases have no symptoms and are only discovered at a routine check-up. Ninety-five per cent of the cases of hypertension have no known cause, but studies show that obesity, stress, faulty diet, the pill, kidney disease and hereditary factors are likely to raise blood pressure. Normal readings are around $\frac{110}{70}/\frac{120}{80}$; in hypertension they may rise as high as $\frac{220}{120}$.

Prevention

Lose weight if you are seriously overweight, and get fit. Take a mild form of exercise: swimming, walking, dancing or yoga. If you have done no exercise for a long time, go gently! Sudden exertion can cause a heart attack, which would rather defeat the purpose of the exercise.

Change your diet: cut out meat, poultry and eggs which are all high in cholesterol. Cut out salt and sugar, which cause water retention and raise blood pressure. Cut down on alcohol and on stimulants such as coffee, tea and cola.

Work at ways to lower stress. In contrast to the popular notion, those most stressed are people who have boring, repetitive and unfulfilling jobs. Poverty, low status, a sense of low self-esteem and poor environmental factors all contribute to stress clearly, changing the outside world is much harder than the inside, although a positive attitude to life is important, as is support and love from family and friends. Many doctors' surgeries and adult education centres run classes in stress management which combine relaxation techniques with breathing exercises.

Treatment

Herbal relaxants

Lavender, melissa, lime flowers, motherwort, skullcap

Plants which lower blood pressure

Hawthorn berries, yarrow, lime blossom

Diuretics (which lower blood pressure by reducing fluid levels in the body)

Dandelion herb, nettles, horsetail.

LOW BLOOD SUGAR (hypoglycaemia)

Again, hypoglycaemia is not life-theatening, unlike hyperglycaemia or diabetes. But it affects countless women's lives. Hypoglycaemia is said to exist when there is too little glucose in the blood stream.

Generally this is not due to an inadequate intake of sugar; in fact usually the reverse is the case. Eating a diet high in sugar and refined carbohydrates causes the pancreas to secrete more insulin than it would normally. This means that the temporary effect of eating a bar of chocolate – increased energy levels – is soon followed by a drop in blood sugar and hence energy. This low level triggers off another craving for sugar, and the whole process is repeated again. A vicious cycle is formed where a woman's blood sugar rises and falls at an alarming rate sometimes causing severe physical and emotional symptoms. These include: lethargy, headaches, drowsiness, irritability and depression (at times severe). Because of the effect it has on the body, sugar can be highly addictive. The body craves more sugar to counteract the tiredness and depression, which in turn causes more tiredness and depression.

Prevention

A high-protein diet provides the right kind of energy for the body and makes the energy levels more stable. Whenever you feel the need for sugar, eat something high in protein, such as cheese, nuts or eggs. It will give you a more sustained boost of energy without triggering a hypoglycaemic reaction. It will take time to educate yourself, as you are weaning yourself off an addictive substance, but eventually the craving will leave you. Sometimes we crave sugar when we want something to drink; remember that sugar retains water in the tissues, so try drinking unsweetened fruit juice or herb tea. Replace white flour bread, cakes, biscuits and cereals with wholemeal products, as these contain some protein and fibre which is digested more slowly thus countering the blood sugar lowering effect. Avoid tea, coffee, alcohol and tobacco which all tend to lower the blood sugar and increase cravings. Liver remedies can help to regulate blood sugar levels: try dandelion root and marigold.

URINARY AND VAGINAL INFECTIONS

CYSTITIS

Cystitis is the inflammation and infection of the bladder. Symptoms vary from the acute – the need to urinate every few minutes, burning pain on passing water, blood or mucus in the urine, fever, back pain, weakness – to the chronic – periodic attacks, with nausea, high fever, burning pain in the bladder, irritability and vomiting.

Cystitis can be caused by a variety of factors: low general health, sexual intercourse, childbirth, irritants such as soaps and vaginal deodorants, bacterial and other infective agents and surgery to the urinary system. Once established, the infection can travel up from the bladder to the kidneys, causing acute back pain, high fever, nausea and vomiting. Left untreated, it can cause permanent damage to the kidneys. Most attacks, however, are mild if very uncomfortable.

Prevention

Never hold on if you need to urinate, as this will stretch the bladder and waste products in the urine will irritate its lining, rendering it more susceptible to infection.

Urinate before and after intercourse.

Ensure personal hygiene by washing frequently and ensure your sexual partner washes his hands and penis before intercourse.

Avoid tampons, vaginal deodorants and panty shields (which all contain perfumes and irritant chemicals), as well as bubble baths, perfumed soaps and douches.

Avoid wearing tight jeans and trousers and try not to wear synthetic underwear. A build-up of heat disposes to infection. Whenever possible, wear skirts without underwear.

Drink lots of liquid (enough to make you urinate 6-8 times daily), but avoid coffee, tea, alcohol and cola as these drinks can irritate the bladder.

Some women say that the diaphragm particularly when used with spermicidal creams, can cause cystitis by pressing on the bladder. Check that the size is correct and try other methods of contraception, preferably condoms, to see if this helps.

TREATMENT

Acute attacks

At the onset of any symptoms, drink as much liquid as you can; barley water is excellent, or pure water and herbal teas. This will dilute the urine, making it less irritating to the bladder, and often this alone will stop an attack. Stop all irritants (see Prevention page 59). Take ½ oz (12.5g) thyme, ½ oz (12.5g) bearberry. Add 1 pint (500ml) boiling water and drink over one day. Repeat until the symptoms go, generally two to three days, and for one extra day. If after seven days there has been no improvement, seek medical advice.

Chronic attacks

Once established, cystitis is hard to eradicate, and prolonged antibiotic therapy, although it stops the symptoms, tends to push the infection deeper into the body and make the bacteria more resistant. Treatment with herbs may take several months but in the end it will heal the bladder and urinary tract, increase resistance and thus eliminate or greatly reduce the frequency and severity of attacks. If this has been a problem for many, many years, the symptoms will not disappear entirely, but with an emphasis on prevention, you will be able to stop a full-blown attack from developing.

Healing remedies

Horsetail, nettles and archangel may be taken in low doses to replace tea and coffee and can be taken indefinitely.

Antiseptics

For short-term use (not more than three weeks at a time): bearberry, thyme and myrrh.

To boost the immune system

Take dandelion, marigold, echinacea, poke root and squaw vine.

THRUSH

Thrush is caused by a yeast fungus, Candida albicans. When the vagina is more acid than normal, the fungus proliferates, causing a white cheesy discharge, redness and irritation, a yeasty smell and occasionally pain on intercourse.

Acidity in the body is caused by antibiotics, the pill, pregnancy, diabetes or a diet high in sugar, carbohydrates, red meat, alcohol, coffee and chemical foods.

A common cause of thrush is antibiotic therapy. Many women will be familiar with this cycle: cystitis attack, antibiotic attack, thrush, anti-fungal remedies, cystitis. Because the urine is more acidic during a bout of cystitis, it predisposes the body to thrush, while the antibiotics kill off the healthy vaginal bacteria which usually keep the fungus at bay. This causes the fungus to proliferate, while at the same time lowers the resistance of the body; thrush then develops, which is treated by anti-fungal agents which further lower the body's resistance, leading back to cystitis. Breaking this unpleasant cycle must begin with the natural treatment of cystitis, which is potentially the more serious of the two, and later tackling the thrush, which may clear up of its own accord once the antibiotic therapy is stopped.

A woman who has repeated attacks of thrush is advised not to use the diaphragm as she may simply reinfect herself each time she uses it. Use sheaths, but avoid spermicides. It is advisable to have her male partner checked to see if he has non-specific thrush or another specially transmitted disease.

Prevention

Cut out sugar from the diet, together with any yeast-based foods such as bread, marmite, beer and fermented foods. Come off the pill, and stop using the diaphragm.

See Prevention of cystitis (page 59) for further details.

Treatment

Acute:
Douche with myrrh and marigold – not more than twice weekly (see Recipe, page 123). Drink archangel and mugwort teas.
Chronic:
Anti-fungal: marigold
For the immune system: marigold and dandelion
As a gynaecological tonic: lady's mantle, mugwort, chaste berry, red clover, poke root and echinacea.

TRICHAMONIASIS

This is a parasite commonly found in both women and men, it is often asymptomatic. When present, the symptoms include a foul-smelling greenish yellow discharge, irritation and sometimes cystitis-like symptoms. It is a sexually transmitted disease and usually men have no symptoms. In one study, it was found that forty per cent of trichamoniasis cases co-existed with gonorrhoea.

Prevention

See Cystitis, page 59. Avoid sharing towels, underwear, flannels and bathing suits.

Treatment:

For the immune system: marigold, dandelion, echinacea and poke root
For gynaecological tonics: myrrh, mugwort, archangel, false unicorn root and squaw vine.

HERPES

Herpes is caused by a virus of which there are two types, I and II. II is generally thought to cause the genital variety of infection. Herpes lesions appear as small blisters or bumps which can be inside the vagina or on the external genitalia, anus or buttocks. Especially during a primary attack the blisters burst, forming small, very painful sores and at this stage they are highly infectious. Enlarged glands, high temperature, secondary infections and a general feeling of malaise can also occur. Before an attack, there is generally an itching feeling on the affected area and often lesions appear in the same place.

Outbreaks occur when the body is stressed, pre-menstrually, after another illness and when the body's immune system is at a low ebb. The first attack is often the most severe; thereafter, attacks may either appear sporadically or with increasing frequency. I have often found a connection with gonorrhoea treated with antibiotics. Other cases seem to have no causative factor, which leads me to suspect that herpes is a systemic disease and not simply a bug which is picked up. Some people are also carriers but have no symptoms. As a virus, herpes is said to be incurable, although some patients have reported no recurrence of their symptoms: long-term studies would be needed to assess this.

Because herpes is stress-related, working at stress reduction can prevent further attacks and reduce their frequency and severity.

Prevention

Avoid stress as far as possible. Learn to worry less and relax more. Over-work, anxiety, exercise, drinking and smoking can all bring on an attack.

Exercise reduces stress and raises the general level of your health. Eat a well-balanced diet low in animal fats, sugar, salt and refined foods.

Use condoms to prevent the spread of herpes and to stop the risk of infection.

As herpes is said to increase the risk of cervical cancer, follow the guidelines in the chapter on Serious diseases (pages 74-76) for cancer prevention.

Treatment

To stimulate the immune system:· marigold, myrrh, dandelion, poke root, echinacea, garlic.
As gynaecological tonics: mugwort, St John's wort, red clover, lady's mantle, false unicorn root.
For use externally: use marigold ointment or lotion on the sores.

Infections of the female reproductive system are notoriously difficult to heal, partly because of its anatomical location. I have found this short visualization helpful especially for women who have had a chronic long standing infection.

Visualization to clear infection

Take yourself to a place where you won't be disturbed for 15-20 minutes. Lie down and make yourself comfortable. Take a few deep breaths and feel your body relaxing into the floor – feel all the tension leaving your body, and be aware that the floor is supporting your weight. Allow your mind to relax downwards – feel it sinking into the floor. Now, cast your mind's eye over your body and see how it looks to you. Are there any 'hot spots', or places where the energy is different? Look for colours and see how they change as you pass over yourself, then imagine white light passing from the crown of your head into your body. Feel it covering every part, all the organs, blood vessels and cells. Feel this white light make all parts of your body equally hot, equally cold. Then imagine a green light passing through you in the same way. Green represents the energy of healing. Check whether there are any areas that need healing and pour extra green light into them. Hold the green light as long as you can inside you and then slowly release it. As it passes out, be aware that it is carrying all the poisons, infections and negative energy out of your body. Slowly come back into the room. It is recommended that you do this meditation daily for at least a week, but preferably for a month or longer.

5 Serious Diseases

PELVIC INFLAMMATORY DISEASE (PID)

IN THE LAST ten years, PID has become increasingly common; the reason for this is unclear, but possible explanations include the increased incidence of sexually transmitted diseases, women having more than one sexual partner and as a consequence of contraception. PID is a chronic condition which, once established, is very difficult to shift. The symptoms vary in each woman but often include the following:

Dull ache in the abdomen
Acute abdominal pain needing hospitalization
Fever which comes and goes
Chills
Lower back or leg pains
Urinary irritation and pain on passing water
Smelly discharge from the vagina
Pain or bleeding during intercourse
Irregular bleeding
Painful periods
Pain mid-cycle (around day 14)
Inflamed cervix, possibly showing up on pap smear
Swollen abdomen
Enlarged lymph nodes
Loss of appetite

Nausea or vomiting
Pain in the liver or kidneys
Spots or rashes on the skin and face
Weakness and depression

Pelvic inflammatory disease occurs when the bacteria have lodged in one or both of the fallopian tubes (salpingitis), the ovaries (oophoritis), both of the above (salpingo-oophoritis) or the uterus (endometriosis). As mentioned above, a common cause is venereal disease, such as gonorrhoea. Other causes include illegally or incompetently performed abortions which result in infection; IUD devices; douching excessively; following childbirth. However, I have also come across cases which seem to have arisen spontaneously with no connection with any of the above.

Generally, the first attack is short and sharp, with acute pain, discharge and fever which responds well to antibiotic therapy. The attacks recur at increasingly closer intervals until several or many of the symptoms are present constantly. Left untreated, PID quickly develops into a chronic persistent condition and has serious complications. Peritonitis is a life-threatening condition where the whole abdominal cavity becomes inflamed, and unless treated speedily, it can be fatal. Other complications of PID include ectopic pregnancy, sterility, miscarriage, infections of the newborn and the increased risk of neonatal death.

The infective agent enters the woman's body during intercourse or after abortion, childbirth, surgery, miscarriage or artificial insemination by donor where the donor has not been screened. It is not uncommon for the male sexual partner of a woman with PID to have no symptoms although he, too, carries the infecting organism. During ovulation, menstruation and childbirth, the cervix is more open than normal, so the risks of infection increase. IUDs also increase the risk, as micro-organisms are able to enter the womb via the string which holds the device in place. Gonorrhoea used to be the commonest cause of PID, but now this has been overtaken by chlamydia and mycoplasma, which are able to live in the vagina for years.

TREATMENT

1. Heat in the form of hot baths, hot pads and hot water bottles definitely relieves the symptoms, but avoid long soaks in the bath after menstruation and ovulation, when the cervix is more open than normal and infection is more likely to occur.
2. Stop using tampons and stop douching, as both can force micro-organisms into the uterus.
3. Always use a barrier method of birth control, such as a condom or the cap, especially during menstruation and ovulation.
4. If you have an IUD, have it removed.
5. Build up your resistance and general level of health. Cut out toxic foods and drinks: additives, colourants, preservatives, preserved meats and poultry, alcohol, tobacco, sugar, tea and coffee, and replace them with lots of wholefoods, fresh foods, fresh fruit and vegetables.
6. Although exercise can be painful once the disease is established, it is very important to keep the circulation to the area dynamic and flowing freely. Tai chi or yoga may well be possible even with the most chronic cases.
7. Herbal treatment has a two-fold approach: local treatment for the uterus itself, and systemic treatment to build up the immune system and enable the body's defence system to fight the infection.

Local remedies

Marigold, lady's mantle, mugwort, blue cohosh, false unicorn root.

Liver remedies to build up the immune system

Marigold, dandelion root, gentian.

Antiseptics to kill the infection

Myrrh, ginger, echinacea, poke root, false unicorn root.

Treatment will necessarily be slow and to begin with may need to be concurrent with antibiotic therapy (particularly if the PID is chronic or there is a risk of peritonitis). With a change in diet and herbal treatment, the condition will slowly begin to improve.

FIBROIDS

Fibroids are non-cancerous (benign) growths found in the uterus. They are very common: 20-30 per cent of all women have fibroids – generally they do not cause any problems, and remain undetected. Usually, they occur in crops, of more than one at a time. They are commoner in younger women and black women, increase in size in pregnancy (oestrogen causes them to do this), and decrease during the menopause. Fibroids are associated with non-ovulatory cycles, where there are low progesterone levels. Symptoms of fibroids vary, but generally speaking they increase bleeding, which can occur both during and between periods. This heavy bleeding necessarily leads to anaemia, and iron levels as low as 4.5mm Hg (the normal level is 10.5mm Hg) have been recorded. Heavy bleeding is the main reason women seek medical advice. Sometimes there is also pain of a cramp-like nature which comes with the periods. There may be pressure symptoms on the bladder, especially if the swellings are large enough to cause an urgency to urinate, incontinence and cystitis-like symptoms. Fibroids can press on the colon, causing constipation, and the small bowel, causing abdominal cramps. They can also be a cause of infertility if they are large enough or numerous enough to fill the uterine cavity.

As stated above, the main problem with fibroids is heavy bleeding. Any bleeding between cycles must first be checked for cancer as this is often the only sign of the disease. Fibroids can be surgically removed, but they tend to grow again. Clearly, the cause of the growth must be ascertained in order for any healing to take place. In my experience, benign growths, wherever they occur in the body, are due to the accumulation of toxins.

TREATMENT

1. Change the diet and eliminate all synthetic and toxic foods and drinks, especially coffee, alcohol, meat and tobacco.
2. Exercise to increase the circulation to the uterus, especially the yoga asanas for pelvic opening and the inverted postures.
3. Herbal treatment is two-fold. Try local treatment to reduce the size of the swellings, with the use of herbal astringents such as shepherd's purse and sage, and the hormonal balancers and gynaecological tonics such as vitex, lady's mantle, false unicorn root, squaw vine and blue cohosh, and circulatory remedies such as yarrow. If the diet has been very toxic, cleanse the liver with a bitter such as dandelion root or marigold.

ENDOMETRIOSIS

Endometriosis is when endometrial tissue (such as that which lines the womb) is found growing outside the uterus. No one is quite sure how this comes about, but there are several factors to be considered.

Firstly, this is a disease of 'civilization', that is to say of the twentieth century. It is commonest in white women who delay child-bearing, begin sexual intercourse late, have low fertility or are sterile. For this reason, it is thought it might have a connection with prolonged ovarian function, that is, menstrual cycles uninterrupted by pregnancy. In countries where women tend to have several children and begin at a young age – China, India, Africa and Latin America – the disease is rare.

There is a theory that instead of flowing out of the womb, blood passes out through the fallopian tubes into the pelvic basin and 'seeds' itself there. Endometrial tissue outside the womb behaves like that within it, in the sense that it has a cycle of increasing and then shedding. It therefore responds to hormonal secretion and declines in pregnancy. It may swell and produce a mass which is thought to be a cancerous growth, but turns out to be endometriosis.

Endometriosis never occurs before puberty, nor after the menopause, and is most common when the hormone secretions are at their height, in the twenties and thirties.

SYMPTOMS

Endometriosis causes menstrual pain, but unlike normal dysmenorrhoea, it occurs one to two days before bleeding starts. It is described as a deep-seated, bearing down kind of pain in the pelvis and vagina, radiating to the back, rectum and thighs.

It generally lasts two to three days, but increases in severity and duration as the disease progresses. Not all women suffer from pain. The first sign may be infertility and endometriosis is discovered on investigation; 15-20 per cent of cases cause infertility. There may also be pain on intercourse, cyclical bowel disturbances, pain on defaecating and rectal bleeding. Urinary symptoms, such as irritation or pain on passing water may also be found.

TREATMENT

One physician recommends that women should have a child every five years to prevent the occurrence of endometriosis. While it is true that pregnancy often clears up the symptoms, it is not a particularly helpful treatment approach. Treatment with progesterone has been found to help as it blocks another hormone (follicle stimulating hormone, or FSH) which increases endometrial tissue. A herbal remedy which has a progesteronal action is vitex and this is to be recommended, together with remedies for the liver, such as dandelion root or marigold, the kidneys, such as horsetail, and yarrow and hawthorn for the circulation. There are several herbal remedies which work like the androgen hormones, blocking the action of FSH, which can be included in a treatment plan; these are sarsaparilla, serenoa and turnera.

Given that the causes are not too clear, treatment is at best speculative. However, as it appears to be a disease of the West, it would be as well to eliminate as many synthetic foodstuffs from the diet as possible, particularly meat, unless it is organically reared, as the synthetic hormones which they invariably contain may be a causative factor.

CANCER

Cancer is such an emotive subject that I really had to think very carefully before entering into such an overheated debate. But I hope what I have written will serve as encouragement to those who are looking for new treatment ideas.

The question I am most frequently asked seems to be whether I have a cure for cancer. People often want to know what will rid themselves of this illness. Given that there is no one cure for any other disease, why should it be that the solution, if it is a solution that we are looking for, is an easy one? Unlikely, given the complexity of the human body, and the complicated combination of factors which lead to the development of any chronic illness. It is estimated that most cancers take twenty years to develop, and that by the time they are detectable, they are well advanced.

So what is cancer? For a variety of reasons, the body begins to grow cells which are abnormal and these cells are stronger, faster-growing and invasive. They gradually replace the healthy cells of the body, taking over some organs which eventually are unable to function properly and begin to atrophy and die. It is usually at this stage that symptoms occur and the cancer can be detected. All types of cancer are different in the rate in which they grow, how they spread and the likelihood of survival or cure.

Generally, cancer is a disease of old age although cervical and lung cancer can happen at any age; it is also a disease of poverty. The poor are more likely to get it than the rich; black women are more susceptible than white women. Bad diet, exposure in the workplace to carcinogenic substances, the prolonged stress of poverty, racial harassment and poor housing all contribute. How, then, can one find a cure? Of course the cure to some extent depends upon changing the nature of society, upon raising the standard of living and ending discrimination. It is less likely to come from any of the wealthy research laboratories supposedly working to that end, as too many livelihoods depend on there not being a cure. However, this is not so helpful if you have discovered a lump in your breast or have an abnormal smear and want to know what you can do about it.

The possible causes of cancer, and therefore its possible prevention and treatment, include the following:

1. Smoking and drinking alcohol. Smoking and drinking heavily account for 20-30 per cent of all cancers.
2. Repeated x-rays.
3. Pollution, and toxic foods such as smoked meats, bacon, additives and refined carbohydrates.
4. High fat consumption.
5. Synthetic hormones, the pill, hormone replacement therapy and the morning after pill have all at some time been implicated in cancers, especially breast cancers. Later studies have cast doubt on these findings, but it does make sense that synthetic hormones should affect breast tissue.
6. Being overweight. Research has found that overweight people (more than 40 per cent) get more cancer and die more frequently from it. In breast cancer there is a connection between high oestrogen levels and of the development of the cancer. It is believed that fat tissue manufactures oestrogens, so try to reduce your weight.
7. Poor diet. Eat a sensible and well-balanced diet, with plenty of whole grains, fruit and vegetables, especially red, yellow and orange vegetables containing vitamin A, which has been found to be a preventative. Eat food high in selenium (eggs, brewer's yeast, mushrooms, tuna, whole grains and brown rice).
8. Stress. Reduce stress levels. Stress is most definitely a cause of cancer and reducing stress can be used successfully in its treatment.

10. Be realistic, and face the truth. You may live a few more years; you may die; or you may live out your natural lifespan. Denial will only send the fears underground and increase your stress levels. It is better to face up to the reality of the situation and if possible have some counselling or therapy to look at the issues in depth.

EARLY DETECTION CONTROVERSY

I come from the generation of women who have been told to have their smears, for whom this test has been made universally available and has been seen as a panacea for the 'problem' of cervical cancer. We have also been told to do breast self-examination monthly after our periods to check for lumps which might be cancerous. However, the statistics for cancer have not changed and appear not to be affected by these early detection methods. Why is this so, and what does it mean?

Given that it can take twenty years for cancer to develop, by the time a lump appears in your breast or you have an abnormal smear, the cancer may be well-established throughout your body. You may have a slow-growing tumour which may take twenty years or more to kill you, or a rapidly-spreading one. The slow-growing type will lie dormant for many years and only in the last two to three years will symptoms become apparent. By then, it is generally too late to do anything. If it is a fast-growing tumour, again there is generally nothing to be done as the tumour will by this stage have spread and it will have affected the whole body.

I was led to believe that cervical cancer was a localized disease and could be cured by local treatment. However, there is growing evidence that it is a systemic condition, and that local surgery will do very little to alleviate the problem. Perhaps, then, early detection is less useful than it has been promoted to be. Why are these yearly and monthly tests performed on women if once the cancer is established, it is too late to act? Statistics are notoriously difficult things to work with or even trust, and cancer statistics are confusing at the best of times: cures are often seen in terms of survival rates of five years or more after the onset of the disease. Personally, I feel that if a woman is unlikely to be interested in any of the medical options offered if cancer were to be diagnosed, there is little point in undergoing the diagnostic tests.

If it is the case that cancer is systemic, then early warning signs will also be systemic. These include fatigue, dull skin and eyes, susceptibility to infections, general low resistance and any chronic condition which does not clear up quickly. At this stage, there is much work that can be done.

1. Change the diet radically and eliminate all toxic foods.
2. Stop smoking and drinking alcohol.
3. Take up some form of exercise, preferably an integrated system such as tai chi or yoga.
4. Examine the amount of stress in your life, and as far as is practical, eliminate it. A short course of counselling or therapy may help to unearth old unresolved conflicts and issues which could be poisoning your system.

TREATMENT

Given that cancers develop at different rates and are detected at different times, it is difficult to give a standard treatment plan. However, following the above guidelines will improve your quality of life and may result in the remission of your cancer. Sometimes, chemotherapy is very effective; at other times, radiotherapy will work, or laser treatment, or diet, or herbs, and occasionally, none of these. Studies of women with breast cancer show that those who are most likely to survive, irrespective of how advanced their disease is, are those who have a good support network, a full and rewarding life, and who are fighters. But again this is not always the case and no real 'recipe' can be given.

The only type of cancer I will discuss here in depth is cervical cancer, as most women have smears which quite often have positive results. The findings for cervical cancer can be classed as follows:

Class CN I: negative
Class CN II: atypical cells but not cancer
Class CN III: atypical cells but suspicious
Class CN IV: probable
Class CN V: definite positive

Cervical cancer is second only to breast cancer in its incidence. It has a clear relation to sexual intercourse, nuns, lesbians and virgins having a negligible incidence. It is believed to be connected to commencing sexual intercourse early in life and having several sexual partners. It is more common in black women, but this has probably more to do with economics than race. Cervical cancer is rarer in Jewish women: this is believed to be because as Jewish men are circumcised, smegma is not allowed to accumulate under the foreskin and cause an infection in the woman. Cervical cancer is also caused by poor hygiene, in particular through male partners not washing properly, chronic cervicitis due to repeated childbirth trauma, and a low general level of health. The herpes virus has been implicated, and in one study 83 per cent of invasive cancer had the herpes virus.

Classes II-IV can also be explained by inflammation and infection. Herbal remedies may be used to clear up the infection locally. I have found a douche of marigold and rosewater most helpful, together with anti-inflammatory remedies such as marigold and cell-building comfrey.

ANTI-CANCER REMEDIES

Again very emotive, but over the years, certain remedies have been found to ease the symptoms of cancer and have a long tradition in its treatment. These include comfrey, red clover, marigold, echinacea and poke root. Newer remedies appear daily and one would need to study the specialist literature carefully before embarking on a course of treatment.

CONCLUSION

It is important to remember to put this disease into context. People die of heart disease and lung disease, but there is no shame involved; people die in accidents and slowly kill themselves with drugs – cancer is another illness and another way to die. Not all heavy drinkers die of alcohol poisoning; not all people with cancer die from cancer. You can reduce the possibilities that you will die from the disease, but more than that no one can do.

We all live in an increasingly polluted world, and it has been estimated that 80 per cent of cancers are due to environmental pollution. Perhaps a better preventative might be to join a lobbying environmental group so that our children can inherit a safer, less carcinogenic planet.

6 Diet and Exercise

CLEARLY, HERBS ARE not miracle workers; they need to be backed up and supported by the lifestyle we choose for ourselves. Both diet and exercise play a vital role in our well-being, and are particularly important with relation to gynaecological issues.

DIET

In recent years, much has been written on the subject of diet, some of it helpful and practical, and some bizarre and harmful. As with all things, common sense, moderation and balance are the key notes for a healthy diet. Extremes of any kind should be avoided, perhaps less for the effect they have on the body than the stress they produce in the psyche. We are designed to be omnivorous beings in the sense that a varied diet is the most suitable for us. We may or may not decide to be vegetarians or vegans, but in any case, we must be sure to choose our diet from the widest range of foods available to us. The macrobiotic adage of only eating the food which grows around us makes some sense, particularly if we translate this to only eating the foods which are in season at a particular time. However, most of us are accustomed to eating exotic foods, which can help vary our diet and supplement our vitamin and mineral intake.

There are many reasons why we should consider looking at our diet. Below are listed illnesses which have been directly linked to eating certain types of foods.

Cancer: too much fat (especially animal fats), lack of fibre.

Benign breast conditions (such as mastitis): too much caffeine.

High blood pressure: too much salt, alcohol and animal fat; too little calcium or potassium.

Heart disease: too many saturated animal fats, cholesterol and sugar; lack of fibre.

Tooth cavities: too much sugar.

Diabetes and hypoglycaemia: too much sugar, lack of fibre.

Osteoporosis: lack of calcium and vitamin D.

Gallstones: lack of fibre.

Bowel disease (diverticulitis, cancer, constipation): lack of fibre.

Obesity: too much fat and sugar; lack of fibre.

GOOD EATING GUIDELINES

1. *Fibre.* This is a very important part of our diet. Fibre is found in whole grains, fruits and vegetables and keeps the whole digestive system healthy. It passes through the body unchanged and acts as a kind of gentle scourer, cleaning and emptying the bowels. Fibre also helps to control the blood sugar levels and so it is essential for the prevention of diabetes and hypoglycaemia. It also keeps down cholesterol. Fibre is filling but not fattening, and so is helpful in obesity and where there are many hungry mouths to feed. Good sources of fibre include potatoes, especially baked or boiled in their skins, peas, beans, lentils, bananas, brown rice, whole grains, swedes and turnips. Fibre can constitute up to 60 per cent of the diet.

2. *Sugar.* Naughty but nice, sugar has been implicated in a wide variety of serious illnesses (see above). In Britain, for example, the average person eats 84 lbs (38kg) of sugar per annum and

30 per cent of adults have none of their natural teeth left and are classified as obese. Try to reduce the sugar intake in your diet to less than ten per cent in the following ways:

i. Check the labels of foods. Ingredients are listed in order of quantity, so if sugar is the first listed, the food contains more of that than anything else. Other names for sugar include corn syrup, lactose, maltose, sucrose, levulose, dextrose, fructose, caramel.

ii. Change from fizzy drinks to pure fruit juices; these can be made fizzy for children by adding mineral water.

iii. In cooking, use honey or molasses; these are far sweeter than sugar so you can reduce the amount used. In any recipe, reduce the amount of sugar stated by half – usually, this does not affect the result.

iv. Switch to sugar-free jams and use concentrated fruit juices to sweeten puddings.

v. Change your breakfast cereal to a low-sugar one like Weetabix or Rice Crispies or better still, make your own muesli sweetened with dried fruits or porridge oats.

vi. Use spices and flavourings to replace sugar, such as cloves, allspice, ginger and vanilla.

3. *Fats.* Again, there has been much publicity about fat consumption – especially animal or saturated fats – in relation to heart disease and hypertension. High fat consumption has also been implicated in certain types of cancers, including breast cancer. Below are some suggestions to reduce fat consumption in the diet.

i. Check the labels of processed foods: avoid animal fat, shortening, tallow lard, hydrogenated oils, corn oil, palm oil.

ii. Eat more fish and poultry and cut down on red meat, bacon and salami. Besides containing high levels of fat, these foods often contain preservatives, pesticides, hormones, antibiotics and other substances fed to animals to increase their weight and profitability.

ii. Substitute low-fat milk, yoghurt and sunflower margarines for milk, cream and butter. Cut down on the amount of hard cheese you eat; if possible, eat fat-reduced cheese or goat's cheese.

iv. Avoid frying foods; grill or bake. If you do fry, use vegetable oils and change the oil each time.

v. Look for low-fat alternatives to dressings and sauces. Tofu mayonnaise, for example, tastes like the real thing but with a much lower fat content.

vi. Buy home-made rather than factory-made cakes and pastries: these are likely to have a lower fat content.

4. *Reduce foods containing cholesterol;* have one egg a day as your daily allowance; reduce offal if eaten.

5. *Reduce salt intake* to 3g daily (the average daily intake is 12g in the UK). Salt is known to contribute to high blood pressure, but also to any kind of water retention – that of PMT, for example, as it puts a strong load on the kidneys. Tips for cutting down on salt include:

    i. Reduce processed foods high in salt such as bacon, salted snacks, nuts, and any food containing monosodium glutamate.

    ii. Do not add salt to food without first tasting it. Try not to add salt whilst cooking.

    iii. Use more herbs and spices in cooking, as they will give the food a strong flavour without requiring the addition of salt.

6. *Reduce your protein intake.* Unless you are pregnant or breastfeeding, protein should only form 12 per cent of the daily diet.

7. *Drink as little alcohol as possible* – one glass of wine daily, one bottle of beer or one measure of spirit.

8. *Eat more vegetarian and less meat-based food.* Vegetarian diets differ – some people call themselves vegetarians when they don't eat meat but eat fish, others (vegans) eat nothing which comes from animals. It really depends on what you feel happiest with. Aside from spiritual practice, most people

become vegetarians because they feel healthier not eating meat and because it is much cheaper. On the other hand, eating meat occasionally cannot be considered harmful. If you are going to eat meat, try to buy organically grown meat which will be free from all the harmful chemicals found in factory farmed meat.

For the newly converted to a vegetarian diet, it is important to be aware of how to combine the food to get whole proteins.

Vegetable proteins are not whole proteins, and cannot be used by the body unless combined in certain ways. For example, rice, whole wheat and potatoes form one class of protein whilst beans, peas and lentils form another. The first category needs to be combined with the second to form a whole protein, for example, rice and beans, peanut butter and bread and potatoes and beans. These whole proteins are absorbed by the body to build tissues and muscles. Food combining may seem complicated; just remember that the starchy foods – rice, bread and potato – need to be combined with the beans. For the newly vegetarian, Indian cookery shows perfectly how food combining works, and there are many good recipe books around.

I do feel it is important to emphasize that we should not attempt to change our diet overnight, nor radically all at once. If you try to do so, you are bound to react emotionally, rather than physically, and then feel angry that you have failed. The aim with a good diet is to eat a reasonably balanced, wide variety of foods. The occasional lapse has no significance and is preferable to carrying a great load of anxiety about your failures.

Most women have a very complicated relationship to food. Many of us have either binged or starved ourselves in reaction to stress. We have been given mixed messages about our bodies and the majority of us imagine ourselves to be too fat, or too curvy, and are worried that we do not fit into the fashion plate ideal. It is vital that we don't use diet as another way to give ourselves a hard time over our bodies. Clearly, the better we eat, the healthier we will be, but emotional factors play as important a role as physical ones and freedom from anxiety is as much to be avoided as pork pies.

EXERCISE

Exercise is another emotive subject, although perhaps less so than diet. All through the book I have emphasized the importance of exercise, and truly it should not be under-estimated. Yet it is also true that those of us who are accustomed to exercise will practise it regularly, whereas those of us who, at school, stood in huddles on windy netball courts will hurriedly turn the page. However, the cult of exercise is growing and the variety of exercises available is wider now than ever. Exercise necessarily involves using the will: not the first time, perhaps, nor the second, but after the novelty wears off, you have to will yourself out of your armchair and out into a drizzling street. When it is cold and you are tired, it is often the last thing that you feel like doing. However, exercise will warm you up and energize you. It will help you lose weight, if that is an aim, and also help you put on muscle tissue if you are too thin. If you smoke and want to give up, you will find it easier to do so and if you are suffering from anxiety or depression, it will leave you with a feeling of well-being.

Generally, though, we only do things because we have to or because someone else is egging us on. If you are planning to begin exercising, try to find a partner to do it with you, so that you can encourage and compete with one another. If you are suffering from an illness, this is the time to begin a gentle form of exercise.

Tai chi or yoga are integrated forms of exercise and as such have much to recommend them.

YOGA

There are several yoga postures which are helpful in gynaecological conditions. Although it is true to say that the whole range of asanas should be practised to gain maximum benefit, still for first aid purposes, or if you are unable to find a teacher, trying some of the following postures over a period of time will be most beneficial.

Inverted postures: head stands and shoulder stands

Both of these postures are excellent for improving the circulation to the pelvis and the legs. Shoulder stands work on the thyroid gland and help with the regulation of hormones; head stands work on the pituitary gland and thus regulate all the hormonal functions in the body. Headstands are stimulating; shoulder stands, relaxing. Do both, but don't try practising head stands alone without shoulder stands in one session; shoulder stands on their own are fine.

Pelvic floor exercises

These are a series of exercises to strengthen the muscles of the pelvis (known as the pelvic floor).

1. They help keep muscle tone in the pelvic area firm so that in pregnancy, the uterus is well supported and the muscles are flexible enough to make childbirth easy; they also speed up healing after childbirth.
2. Where there is urinary incontinence, they strengthen the muscles of the bladder and aid in control of urination.
3. Where there is constipation due to weak muscles, they improve muscle tone and make bowel movements easier.
4. Where there is prolapse, they firm up the tissues.

The muscle action involves lifting the pelvic muscles which control the pelvic and urinary muscle openings. Next time you are urinating, try to stop the flow in mid-stream. It is these muscles you will be working with.

Lying down, contract the muscles and hold them in for three seconds. Repeat this five times. During the day (at any time, you don't have to lie down for this), repeat until you can do ten groups of five.

Imagine that you are tightening the muscles while climbing upwards slowly. Go up in stages. Hold at the top and come down slowly again.

Imagine that you are sucking air or water into your vagina. Repeat five times. Do 5-6 times daily.

VITAMINS AND MINERALS

	ACTIONS	SOURCES
Vitamin A	Helps prevent infection. Helps to improve blindness. Strengthens skin, lungs, bones and teeth.	Fish-liver oil, tuna, milk, butter, egg yolk, cheese, dark green and yellow vegetables and fruits.
Vitamin D	Regulates calcium and phosphorus absorption for strong bones and teeth.	Sunlight on bare skin, fish liver oils, tuna.

Vitamin E	Stabilizes tissues; especially useful for circulatory and heart tissue.	Vegetable oils, soya, wheat germ, wheat, brown rice, legumes, egg yolk.
Vitamin B1	For nerves, energy, good digestion.	Wholegrain bread, cereals, yeast, wheat germ.
Vitamin B12	Needed for protein, fat and carbohydrate metabolism.	Comfrey, peas, beans, nuts.
Vitamin C	Holds cells together, helps wounds heal, aids iron absorption.	Green leafy vegetables, fruit.
Calcium	Strengthens bones, teeth, nerves and muscles, helps blood clotting.	Milk and milk products, leafy greens, molasses, sesame seeds, tofu, cashew nuts.
Phosphorus	Metabolizes fats and carbohydrates. With calcium, forms strong bones and teeth.	Milk, cheese, eggs, nuts and seeds, legumes, whole grains.
Magnesium	Improves carbohydrate metabolism, muscle and nerve tissue.	Wholegrains, leafy greens, beans, nuts.
Potassium	For healthy nerves and muscles.	Bananas, potatoes, dark leafy greens, peanut butter, molasses, milk.

| Sodium | Regulates fluid levels balance between sodium and potassium is important. | Table salt, seaweeds. |
| Iron | Essential for red blood cells and therefore carrying oxygen around the body. | Molasses, miso, apricots, dandelions, yeast, wholegrains. |

7   The Herbal

I HAVE CHOSEN the following herbs because they are the ones that I have used the most in my practice which I like and with which I feel an affinity. I have what is considered in some circles a rather unorthodox relationship to plants: I see each plant very much as an individual, with a character, likes and dislikes, affinities and aversions. Some plants will work for some people and not for others. I discovered this rather startling fact many years ago when doing my clinical training. Twice I had very spectacular results with a remedy and in my excitement I encouraged a fellow student to try the same plant on a similar patient. The remedy which worked so well for me and my patient had no effect at all on the patient of my colleague.

I could not understand it, but put it down to my ignorance, or something I didn't yet understand. Later on, the same thing happened again. And I decided something strange was going on. I had thought of the plants as being neutral; dandelion was good for the livers; any liver. Later, when I began my more in-depth work with plants, I understood why this had happened. Each plant has a very clear and often very strong personality. Certain plants have a great affinity with some people, but an aversion to others. For example, as much as I extol the virtue of dandelion, I cannot take the stuff myself. I drop the bottle, spill the tincture, leave it on buses and do everything rather than take it, because I know that constitutionally it does not suit me.

I think this explains why some people have spectacular results with herbal remedies and others none at all. How do you tell which remedy is applicable to you, and what will suit you? The best way, once you have narrowed down the remedies which will heal the physical condition you have, is to read the emotional descriptions carefully and find one which fits in best with the way you are feeling. I do not wish to categorize the plants rigidly or extensively, as in homoeopathy, because I feel very strongly that we should not define them too exactly. We can set loose parameters within which to explore a remedy and its actions but we must remain flexible and open-minded, never thinking we have found out all there is to know.

In the physical applications of the plant, rather than listing endless actions I have restricted myself to those actions pertinent to gynaecology or conditions affecting the reproductive system. The list of plants in this herbal is not exhaustive, as I feel it is better to have less information and use it well than to have too much and become confused.

Archangel

Lamium album

PART USED:	whole herb
PICKING TIME:	June–September
MAIN ACTIONS:	haemostatic, diaphoretic, astringent, blood purifier, sedative
CONSTITUENTS:	tannin, saponins, mucilage, essential oil
COMMON NAMES:	white dead nettle, blind nettle, deaf nettle, dumb nettle

PHYSICAL USES

Archangel is an astringent, and is used to stop bleeding or to reduce heavy menstrual blood loss. This is a particularly useful herb in puberty, when there is often heavy and irregular bleeding. It is most helpful for non-specific discharges or leucorrhoea, and can be used for painful and irregular periods. It is a blood purifier, which means that it has a generalized cleansing action on the body and is particularly useful for acne and pimples. It is a general gynaecological tonic and can be used where there is weakness, anaemia, low blood pressure or general debility. It has a mild tranquillizing effect.

A tonic for puberty

1 oz (7g) yarrow
1 oz (7g) archangel
1 pint (500ml) water

Pour the boiling water on the plants and let stand for 15 minutes. Take a wineglassful three times daily.

A douche for leucorrhoea (non-infective discharge, white in colour)

1 oz (25g) archangel
1 pint (500ml) water

Make tea from the plant in the usual way and then boil to reduce the liquid to ⅓ pint (170ml). Add an equal amount of rosewater. Dose: 1 tablespoon of the mixture diluted in warm water. Use once daily as a douche, or wash the genitalia with the mixture to soothe itching and irritation.

Facial wash for acne, blackheads and spotty skin

3 fl oz (80ml) rose water or orange flower water
⅓ fl oz (10ml) tincture of archangel
⅓ fl oz (10ml) tincture of marigold

Mix well and bottle. After cleansing the skin, dab on the lotion with cotton wool to dry up spots and oily skin.

EMOTIONAL USES

Archangel is a herb of youth – it has a flavour of innocence about it. It stands for cleanness, brightness, purity and wholesomeness. It has a revitalizing action on the psyche and is especially useful for women who have lost their innocence. Perhaps it is most helpful after rape or sexual trauma, after abortion or any emotional experience which has taken some of the lightness away. It is good for people who are severely depressed, who have lost hope, feel there is no light and have forgotten how to find joy.

Bearberry

Arctostaphylos uva ursi

PART USED:	leaves
PICKING TIME:	June–September
MAIN ACTIONS:	antiseptic, astringent, tonic, analgesic
CONSTITUENTS:	glycosides, tannin, flavonoids
COMMON NAMES:	bear's grape, arbutus

PHYSICAL USES

Bearberry is a powerful and effective urinary antiseptic. It is the herb of choice for cystitis, urinary incontinence and blood in the urine. It has a heating action for chills in the kidney and bladder: it tones the whole urinary system and stimulates the blood flow to that area. It increases the effectiveness of the kidneys and thus the excretion of waste products from the body. Bearberry can also be used for the treatment of kidney stones, gravel, urethritis and nephritis. It works best when the urine is alkaline, which is usually true of vegetarians: carnivores should take bicarbonate of soda to make it more effective. It has a slight pain-killing action which is also helpful in painful urinary diseases. It can be used in the treatment of arthritis associated with kidney imbalance. As a strong astringent, it helps reduce heavy bleeding from the womb, discharges and haemorrhoids.

Mixture for cystitis

1 oz (25g) bearberry leaves
1 oz (25g) thyme herb
2 pints (1 litre) boiling water

Add the boiling water to the herbs, cover and let stand for 20 minutes. Drink during the course of 48 hours. Repeat until symptoms disappear. Do not take for more than 21 days.

EMOTIONAL USES

I associate bearberry with anger – anger expressed, or anger suppressed and experienced as depression. Usually there are great passions boiling away which erupt from time to time or are channelled or suppressed by alcohol, food or drugs. Bearberry helps to find a safer way to express these feelings, and to let off steam. In women, there is often high energy which has been repressed for many years, a good deal of vitality has been hidden because it was experienced as too much. That energy has gone inwards and tends to be expressed as self-destruction, negativity and hopelessness. Bearberry will help to get this energy moving again, allowing the woman to find her inner source of power, her life energy.

Blue Cohosh

Caulophyllum thalictroides

PART USED:	root
PICKING TIME:	autumn
MAIN ACTIONS:	reproductive tonic, anti-spasmodic
CONSTITUENTS:	alkaloids, saponins

PHYSICAL USES

Blue cohosh is a tonic to the whole reproductive system and can be used where there is congestion and weakness. It will bring on delayed periods and helps to regulate the menstrual cycle and to relieve period pains. Use for chronic conditions such as fibroids, endometriosis and pelvic inflammatory disease. It is a useful remedy to help conception occur if there has been difficulty conceiving. It has been used for threatened miscarriage, and taken during the last month to ease the birth.

To strengthen the uterus, blue cohosh combines well with yarrow and motherwort.

EMOTIONAL USES

For people who through life's traumas have become hard and brittle; for meanness, envy, jealousy, the very worst of human feelings. For cruelty, to open the heart, to soften anger and the passions generally. It has a calming, soothing, warming and lightening effect. Take as a tea or tincture nightly before sleeping.

Chamomile

Anthemis nobile

PART USED:	flowers
PICKING TIME:	July–August
MAIN ACTIONS:	antispasmodic, relaxant, bitter, digestive, antiseptic
CONSTITUENTS:	volatile oil, bitter, valerianic acid, flavonoids
COMMON NAMES:	maythen (saxon), manzanilla

PHYSICAL USES

A gentle sedative and muscle relaxant, chamomile is an excellent gynaecological remedy. Use to ease painful periods, premenstrual headaches and tension before the period. It relaxes the body, irons out any muscle spasms and allows the menstrual blood to flow freely. I have found chamomile especially useful for puberty and the menopause, when there is anxiety, palpitations, insomnia and general hyperactivity. It has a gentle warming action on the whole body. Chamomile is especially good for the skin used externally as a wash or as an internal medicine. Use for acne, pimples and blackheads. It is an antiseptic and can be used in combination with other remedies for any infection.

Relaxing tea for headaches and insomnia

½ oz (25g) chamomile flowers
½ oz (25g) melissa flowers

Make the tea in the usual way, allow to stand and sip slowly.

Facial wash for pimples, acne etc.

½ oz (25g) chamomile flowers
1 pint (500ml) water

Bring the mixture to the boil, simmer gently for 10 minutes. Strain and cool. Dab on the skin 2-3 times daily.

EMOTIONAL USES

Use chamomile where there is fear and anxiety, or for someone who is oversensitive, touchy or nervous. It relaxes and grounds the person, making her feel stronger and more able to withstand shocks and trauma. When there are panic attacks and acute anxiety, a few drops of the tincture or a warm tea will have a relaxing and calming effect. Use when someone seems angry, but her anger is based on fear rather than rage.

Cleavers

Galium aparine

PART USED: whole herb
PICKING TIME: all summer
MAIN ACTIONS: blood cleanser, demulcent, diuretic
CONSTITUENTS: silica, tannin
COMMON NAMES: goosegrass, hedgeriff, robin-run-in-the-
                     grass, everlasting friendship

PHYSICAL USES

Cleavers works on the immune system, cleansing and unclogging the body. Use wherever there is water retention, oedema, swollen ankles and fingers. I have found it especially useful for PMT, where the body can feel waterlogged and sluggish: it works to get the system moving again, to expel the excess water and stimulate the metabolism. Where there is overweight due to fluid retention and slow metabolism, cleavers is most useful. It is a diuretic and stimulates the action of the kidneys. Use for cystitis, kidney stones and urethritis. It has an affinity for breast tissue and will help alleviate lumps in the breast, mastitis and swollen, painful breasts. As a blood cleanser, cleavers is used to treat a variety of skin diseases: acne, eczema and psoriasis. Because it is a deep-acting remedy, it needs to be taken over a period of several months before a substantial change is seen.

Mixture for acne:

1 part cleavers
1 part marigold
1 part comfrey

Combine either as a herbal tea (½ oz mixed herbs to 1 pint water) or in a tincture and take for 1-3 months, three times daily.

EMOTIONAL USES

Cleavers is calming and yet invigorating. It helps to settle the emotions after a shock or when a great change is about to happen. For this reason it is to be recommended for women at the menopause to ease the transition that is the change of life. It provides an emotional breathing space, a hiatus in the midst of a hectic, busy life. Use for those whose lives are full, but who perhaps lack serenity or who need another perspective on life.

Comfrey
Symphytum officinale

PART USED: leaves, flowers and roots

PICKING TIME: leaves and flowers June–September,
roots November and March

MAIN ACTIONS: wound healing, soothing, tissue building,
nutritive

CONSTITUENTS: allantoin, tannins, gum, resin, alkaloids,
mucilage, vitamin B12

COMMON NAMES: knitbone, boneset, blackwort, bruisewort,
consolida, ass' ear

PHYSICAL USES

Leaves and flowers: These are soothing, healing and relaxing for the urinary and reproductive systems. Comfrey is cooling to the kidneys and bladder, and is useful for cystitis where there is pain and irritation. Use if there is a discharge which feels hot and itchy and for excessive blood loss. Allantoin has been found to heal all types of tissue but has a special affinity for bones, muscles and ligaments. Used in any diseases of these parts, comfrey is especially helpful for brittle bones, both as a treatment and as a preventative. It can also be used in chronic skin disease, such as acne, eczema and psoriasis, to heal the skin tissue. The flowering tops of the comfrey plant contain vitamin B12, which is needed by all vegans. Chop the leaves and flowers and add to soups and salads. Comfrey is helpful to 'build the blood'. Use where there is heavy bleeding to avoid the possibility of anaemia and for its treatment. Traditionally comfrey was used to treat growths.

Root: The root contains a great deal of mucilage which is used to soothe and heal inflamed tissue. Use where there has been infection or inflammation. Traditionally used for stomach ulcers, bronchitis and cystitis, comfrey is also helpful for infections in the womb such as PID and in the treatment of discharges.

A blood tonic for weakness and anaemia

1 part comfrey
1 part nettle
1 part dandelion root
1 part horsetail

Take either in the form of a tea (½ oz mixed herbs to 1 pint water) or as a tincture.

EMOTIONAL USES

Comfrey assists healing after profound emotional shock, grave illnesses or despair, and grounds and centres the psyche. Use where the person feels scattered and fragmented and needs to gather her forces again. Comfrey helps to create structure and form in lives that are disorganized or chaotic. Solidifying, stabilizing, calming, comfrey is an excellent remedy for the bereaved.

Cramp Bark   *Viburnum opulus*

PART USED: the bark
PICKING TIME: April and May
MAIN ACTIONS: anti-spasmodic, astringent, sedative
CONSTITUENTS: bitters, valerianic acid, tannin

PHYSICAL USES

This is an excellent remedy for pain and muscle spasm. It relaxes
the muscles in the uterus and is therefore the remedy of choice
for painful periods; it can also be used in threatened miscarriage.
It helps to relieve excess blood loss and heavy bleeding during
the menopause.

Combine with false unicorn root for painful periods.

EMOTIONAL USES

Cramp bark gives the emotions a flexibility; it helps to relax mental
rigidity and conformity in people who cling, who won't let people
and situations go, who hold on because they have a need to control
and to dominate. It allows the person to relax and open out, to
be more willing to accept the point of view of others, and to be
more self-reliant so that her energy or sense of power resides
within her and is not focused in other people. Take the remedy
as a tea in the normal way.

Dandelion

Taraxacum officinalis

PART USED:	root, leaves and flowers
PICKING TIME:	root: November to March; flowers/leaves: May–September
MAIN ACTIONS:	liver tonic, healing, diuretic, digestive stimulant
CONSTITUENTS:	potassium, bitter principles, tannin
COMMON NAMES:	piss-in-the-bed, dent de lion, devil's milk pail, priest's crown

PHYSICAL USES

Root: the root is used mainly for the liver. It is used for all liver diseases: hepatitis, cirrhosis, jaundice, chronic liver congestion. Use wherever there is poor digestion, bloating after meals, swollen abdomen, constipation or flatulence. It is an excellent remedy for varicose veins and haemorrhoids. Use in PMT and wherever the hormones are imbalanced, the cycle irregular or the bleeding abnormal. As a liver remedy, Dandelion assists the body's immune system and is therefore used whenever there are infections or viruses or the person is run down and debilitated. Use dandelion to regulate the blood sugar levels of the body, hypoglycaemia and in PMT where this is a problem. It can be used as a deep-acting blood purifier for skin conditions like acne and eczema.

Flowers and leaves: these have a stronger action on the kidneys. Dandelion is a powerful diuretic, so much so it has to be used with care with those suffering from low blood pressure as it might lower it further. It is therefore an excellent remedy for high blood pressure, especially as it contains potassium, which is lost from the body when one uses chemical diuretics. Use in water retention, oedema and for the symptomatic relief of PMT. Dandelion is used in the treatment of cystitis, kidney stones and gravel.

EMOTIONAL USES

Dandelion is a liberator of anger and is especially useful for people who are servers of others, such as mothers of small children, nurses, social workers and other carers: in short, people whose major focus in life is the care of those less able to defend themselves. While these are good and noble works, often such people have not had much choice, as in the case of carers, or have now become resentful of the load that is put on their shoulders. They cannot hit out at those they care for, and often they receive a lot of approval from those around them and feel unable to express resentments or make demands. The anger builds up, and perhaps they become depressed or develop physical stress symptoms such as stomach ulcers or colitis. In either case, there is a blockage of the emotions, a build-up of tension and a sense of pressure in the body. Dandelion will help to relieve that pressure and give the opportunity to express some of these feelings. Often this takes the form of 'blowing one's top', which often happens when taking dandelion and other liver remedies. However, this release of pressure creates space into which other, more sustaining energies can develop, allowing for greater assertion and more self-expression.

Echinacea

Echinacea angustifolia

PART USED:	the root
PICKING TIME:	autumn
MAIN ACTIONS:	antiseptic, anti-microbial
CONSTITUENTS:	volatile oil, resin, insulin, sucrose

PHYSICAL USES

Echinacea stimulates the body's immune system and helps combat all types of infections, bacterial and viral. Use for herpes, trichamoniasis, chronic cystitis and especially for PID. It stimulates the excretion of toxins from the body and helps to build up resistance to infection. Use for chronic cystitis, PID and herpes. DO NOT TAKE DURING PREGNANCY.

EMOTIONAL USES

This remedy gives strength and light and hope in times of great distress and trauma. It brings the qualities of lightness, optimism and gaiety, and gives freedom from care, burdens and pessimistic thoughts. Conversely, it is a useful remedy for people who are unrealistically optimistic, people who won't deal with reality as it is and escape at the first opportunity.

Take the tea or 5 to 10 drops of the tincture three times daily, when there is a crisis for as long as there is a need; for grounding, take the normal dose.

False Unicorn Root   *Chamaelirium luteum*

PART USED:	the root
PICKING TIME:	autumn
MAIN ACTIONS:	tonic to the uterus, diuretic
CONSTITUENTS:	saponins

PHYSICAL USES

False unicorn root contains substances (saponins) which are similar to oestrogen (female hormone). It is a healing restorative to the reproductive system, and harmonizes the periods, especially where there is heavy bleeding and a feeling of heaviness and bloating in the uterus. Use for discharges, also where the periods are irregular and there is pain with menstruation. It is used in the treatment of infertility and can be taken during the last month of pregnancy to ease childbirth. Use as a tonic in the treatment of pelvic inflammatory disease (PID).

EMOTIONAL USES

This is an ideal remedy for people who fear they have a serious illness, like cancer; and helps cope with the fear of death and dying, of decay, the obsession with bodily functions, sickness and death. It is also good for hypochondria and for those recovering from a serious illness who need to leave those symptoms behind, and make a new start emotionally as well as physically. Take the medicine as a tea in the usual manner.

Garlic

Allium sativum

PART USED:	the bulb
PICKING TIME:	autumn
MAIN ACTIONS:	antiseptic, antiviral, diaphoretic, cholagogic, hypotensive, antispasmodic, antimicrobial
CONSTITUENTS:	volatile oil, mucilage, sulphur, vitamins C, A and B, hormonal-type substances, iodine
COMMON NAMES:	poor man's treacle, ajo

PHYSICAL USES

Garlic is a powerful antiseptic and can be used in lung infections (bronchitis), kidney and bladder infections (cystitis, nephritis), infections in the uterus (PID) and discharges in general. It is anti-fungal and therefore is very helpful in thrush, antiseptic and so can be used in trichamoniasis, and as an anti-viral for use in herpes, post-viral syndrome and bronchitis. It stimulates liver function and the action of the gall bladder, so can be used in PMT and other hormonally based conditions. It lowers the blood pressure, is said to lower blood cholesterol and is recommended for arteriosclerosis and other vascular diseases, such as angina, poor circulation and Reynaud's disease. It is hot and spicy, so don't use it where the stomach is inflamed, or where there has been gastritis or stomach ulcers.

Recipe for thrush: garlic pessary

Carefully peel one clove of garlic, taking care not to cut into the pulp. Wrap it in bandage gauze and insert into the vagina. Change every 6-8 hours. It cannot get lost in the vagina, as the opening of the cervix (into the womb) is about the size of a pinhead, far too small for anything except liquid to pass through.

EMOTIONAL USES

Hot and fiery, garlic helps to localize the fire element which is so easily lost in damp temperate climates: fire, passion, energy and vigour – the energy that children have in abundance, which bit by bit is socialized out of them. Garlic helps the playful part of ourselves, impish, energized, even wild. Use for those who are burdened down by life, who are serious, dutiful, boring; for earth-bound types who could do with a little spice, a little excitement. Also for women who are fiery in nature and perhaps have lost it temporarily, through depression, illness or cultural dislocation.

Gentian Root

Gentiana lutea

PART USED:	the root
PICKING TIME:	autumn
MAIN ACTIONS:	bitter tonic, digestive stimulant
CONSTITUENTS:	bitter principles, tannin, mucilage

PHYSICAL USES

Gentian is a powerful liver remedy and should be avoided if there is any debility. It stimulates the liver to de-toxify the body and is therefore an excellent remedy for pre-menstrual tension, infections of the reproductive system and for venereal disease. As it stimulates the digestion, use for loss of appetite, dyspepsia, flatulence, and poor digestion. It can be used in the long-term treatment of depression and migraine.

EMOTIONAL USES

For depression due to the suppression of anger and resentment; lethargy, apathy, tearfulness, pessimism or self-hatred. Gentian helps to open up the emotions so that the anger can be expressed. Often after taking this remedy, the patient feels angry a lot of the time, but this stage passes quickly and she begins to feel calmer and more in her own power than before; and less of a victim.

Take a few drops of the tincture (the tea is very bitter) each morning before facing the day.

Ginger

Zingiberis officinalis

PART USED: rhizome
PICKING TIME: all year
MAIN ACTIONS: stimulant, digestive, carminative,
    diaphoretic, sedative
CONSTITUENTS: volatile oil, alkaloids, resins

PHYSICAL USES

Being a hot herb, ginger is useful to relax tense muscles. I use it to relieve muscle spasms in period pain; it also relaxes the system generally. It helps those who suffer from poor circulation, low blood pressure, dizziness or chilblains, and those who feel the cold badly. Ginger is helpful for those who feel weak and debilitated and feel they need extra blood in their bodies and can be used in the treatment of headache, catarrh and sinus problems. It reduces water retention in the body by increasing sweating.

Recipe for period pain

½ oz (25g) ginger root
½ oz (25g) yarrow

Chop the ginger and mix with the yarrow. Make the tea in the normal way. Sweeten with honey and sip slowly.

EMOTIONAL USES

Ginger warms the feelings as well as the body. Use for people who are frozen emotionally, whether through fear or numbness after shock; for those who are cool and aloof who find it hard to relate to others. Ginger warms the heart and allows for an easing of tension, a relaxing and opening out.

Hawthorn

Crategus oxycanthoides

PART USED:	the berries
PICKING TIME:	autumn
MAIN ACTIONS:	sedative, circulatory remedy
CONSTITUENTS:	rutin, bioflavonoids, tannins
COMMON NAMES:	May blossom, quickthorn, whitethorn, haw, pixie pears, cuckoo beads, chunky cheese, lady's meal

PHYSICAL USES

Hawthorn is the main remedy for the heart and the circulation. Use wherever there are problems with the circulation; high blood pressure, low blood pressure, heart disease, palpitations, hot flushes, varicose veins, coronary heart disease, angina. It has a sedative action and is especially useful where the high blood pressure is stress-related. It is a useful remedy for improving the circulation to the uterus in chronic conditions, like fibroids, endometriosis and PID.

EMOTIONAL USES

As well as being a physical heart remedy, hawthorn also works on the emotional heart. Use for people who find it hard to express their emotions, be they angry or loving. There has been found to be a connection with physical heart conditions and the inability to relate emotionally. In our culture, we are not encouraged to express our feelings – it is more acceptable to remain cool and logical and not to rant and rave. From a health point of view this is a disaster as the feelings are there anyway, whether they are expressed or not. Buried anger, resentment and hurt feelings easily turn into bitterness and resentment. Hawthorn is good for those who feel life has been hard, that they have had more than their fair share of disappointments and of pain.

Horsetail

Equisetum arvensis

PART USED:	whole plant
PICKING TIME:	June, July
MAIN ACTIONS:	diuretic, nutritive, healing, astringent
CONSTITUENTS:	silica, saponins, flavonoids, alkaloids
COMMON NAMES:	mare's tail

PHYSICAL USES

Rich in nutrients, horsetail is used to build up the blood, to re-mineralize it. Use in anaemia, when there is heavy blood loss, at puberty and the menopause when the body is changing rapidly and needs extra nutrition. Especially good for bone tissue, horsetail is the best remedy for brittle bones, for arthritis and rheumatism. Horsetail is also astringent and so will help to reduce heavy blood loss and vaginal discharges. It tones up muscle tissue and is used for urinary incontinence and uterine prolapse. Because of its mineral content, horsetail is also used to repair brittle and damaged hair and nails and to heal the skin; use with other remedies for the treatment of acne.

An antiseptic, horsetail is used for the kidneys and bladder and is especially useful in cystitis where there is bleeding. Horsetail is one of the remedies which helps to regulate the sugar in the blood stream and is useful for low blood sugar and PMT.

Recipe to strengthen the bones

Mix together equal parts: horsetail
nettle
comfrey
dandelion root

Make up either as a tea or a tincture. Take daily for 2-3 months.

For prolapse

Mix together equal parts: horsetail
  sage
  shepherd's purse
  mugwort

Make up as a tea (½ oz herbs to 1 pint of water) and douche (undiluted but strained) once daily. Try to retain the liquid as long as possible.

EMOTIONAL USES

Just as horsetail strengthens the bones physically and makes them less brittle, so it makes the emotions more pliable and more elastic. A horsetail type tends to be cold, aloof, sometimes aggressive and hostile. They are unbending, stubborn, difficult and find it hard to be flexible, to meet situations and people halfway. With great will-power and stamina, they are often hard workers and expect a lot from those around them. Perfectionists, they are frequently disappointed in people but hide their hurt behind a stern façade.

Lady's Mantle   *Alchemilla vulgaris*

PART USED: flowers and leaves
PICKING TIME: June/July
MAIN ACTIONS: astringent, healing, gynaecological tonic
CONSTITUENTS: tannin, bitters, salicylic acid
COMMON NAMES: alkmelych (alchemy)

PHYSICAL USES

Lady's mantle is an excellent gynaecological remedy, and can be
used for a wide variety of conditions. It is a tonic and hormonal
regulator and it gently balances and harmonizes the menstrual
cycle. Use in amenorrhoea, where the menses have stopped for
one reason or another, and for irregular cycles in puberty, at the
onset of the menopause or whenever they occur. Taken for 2-3
months, lady's mantle will rebalance the hormones in severe PMT.
If a woman is suffering from a variety of symptoms at the
menopause and is contemplating HRT, take this remedy for 2-3
months and the problems should clear up. Use for chronic period
pains, migraine or acne associated with the menses, thrush or
other vaginal infections to regulate the hormone secretions. In
severe conditions, always include lady's mantle as a gentle but
effective balancer. Use where there has been trauma to the uterus;
miscarriage, abortion, IUD insertion, PID or any kind of surgery.

EMOTIONAL USES

Lady's mantle is one of what I call the flying herbs. By this I don't
mean that you can get on your broomstick and head for the hills,
but that it lifts the spirits, widens the horizons, expands

possibilities, and opens up vistas. Its name, *alchemilla*, suggests that it is an alchemical plant, that it transforms. Use for people who are stuck, who feel in a rut, earthbound, bored, uninspired. It can help you to make changes, break ties and move on in your life.

Lavender
Lavendula officinalis

PART USED:	flowers
PICKING TIME:	June–August
MAIN ACTIONS:	sedative, antiseptic, antispasmodic
CONSTITUENTS:	volatile oil, bitter
COMMON NAMES:	The name lavender comes from the Latin, *Lavare*, to wash; it is also called elf leaf, nard, asarum

PHYSICAL USES

A strong relaxing herb, lavender is a tonic to the nervous system. It is healing and strengthening to nervous tissue. Use for anxiety, nervousness, anxiety headaches, insomnia, migraine, palpitations. It lowers high blood pressure which is caused by stress, calms a racing heart and reduces hot flushes brought on by anxiety: it can be used as a first-aid remedy in a panic attack. Lavender has a stimulating action on the liver and so helps digestive problems due to tension and anxiety; it reduces a feeling of bloating after meals, constipation or flatulence. It is helpful for dizziness and fainting attacks as well as for travel sickness.

A nerve tonic and relaxant

lavender
rosemary
dandelion root

Mix in equal proportions, either as a tea (½ oz mixed herbs to 1 pint water) or a tincture. Take twice daily for 3-4 weeks.

EMOTIONAL USES

Lavender helps to protect and filter emotional energies entering the psyche. Some people are far more sensitive than others and feel almost battered by the sensory impressions they take in. These people are often psychic and react badly to loud noises, discord, ugliness and aggression. Although sensitivity in itself is no bad thing, we nevertheless need to live in this world. Lavender helps a person to be able to protect herself better, so that she feels less vulnerable and less jarred by everyday living.

Lime Blossom   *Tilia europea*

PART USED: flowers
PICKING TIME: June–July
MAIN ACTIONS: sedative, diaphoretic, circulatory remedy
CONSTITUENTS: volatile oil, mucilage, tannin, saponins

PHYSICAL USES

Lime flowers are a strong sedative and as such should be used
with respect and caution. Excellent in cases of severe insomnia,
panic attacks and anxiety, for the symptomatic treatment of
migraine and for any pain. Use alongside other remedies for PID,
endometriosis, and cramps; it is an excellent pain reliever. Lime
flowers also work on the circulation. Traditionally they were used
as a preventative for arteriosclerosis, to reduce blood cholesterol
and equalize or normalize the circulation. Use in severe cases of
high blood pressure, especially where stress is believed to be a
major cause. Lime blossom can be used to wean women off
tranquillizers and barbiturates gradually, minimizing the
withdrawal symptoms.

EMOTIONAL USES

A remedy for those who need more love in their lives, who find
it hard to receive love, to express love. Such people may have been
damaged as children, suffered cruelty at the hands of others;
perhaps they have had traumatic experiences in relationships or
been abused. They hide their vulnerability behind a mask of
coldness and indifference, but they are highly sensitive. Lime
blossom is for those who are givers, but find it hard to receive;

for those who seem cut off from warmth, who are distant, who are difficult to reach. It softens, warms and helps build trust and a willingness to open up to others.

Marigold

Calendula officinalis

PART USED:	flowers
PICKING TIME:	August
MAIN ACTIONS:	hepatic, healing, astringent, gynaecological tonic
CONSTITUENTS:	bitter, saponins, sterols, mucilage, gum
COMMON NAMES:	calendula, golds, ruddes, mary gowles, marygold

PHYSICAL USES

Marigold has to be my favourite plant, not only because it is so good to look at but because it is a veritable pharmacy in its own right. I could probably write a book on this plant alone, but will endeavour to restrict myself to the most relevant facts.

For the liver, marigold is the remedy par excellence; also for congestion, jaundice, cirrhosis, poor digestion, constipation and wind. It is a healing remedy for the veins, and is used for varicose veins, haemorrhoids and to improve the circulation to the pelvis generally. Because of its liver function, marigold is used for PMT to regulate the hormone levels in the blood stream, cleanse the blood and control the absorption of nutrients. It regulates the menstrual cycle, so use both in puberty and at the menopause. It reduces cysts, polyps, breast swellings, lumps and any unusual growths. It is a powerful healing agent and is the remedy of choice in PID, after abortion, miscarriage or any other trauma. It is anti-fungal and is therefore used to treat thrush, both externally as a douche and internally. Use for discharges, problems with the cervix, and after abnormal smears, erosions and tears. Marigold is a stimulant of the immune system and can therefore be used in any infection where there is debility or weakness, and after viral attacks, swollen lymph glands or herpes. It has a hormonal action, so use in endometriosis and in the menopause for vaginal dryness. It is also a remedy for the skin, working through the liver and the lymphatic system. Use for acne, eczema and teenage spots.

Douche for thrush

½ oz (25g) marigold flowers
½ oz (25g) mugwort
1 pint (500ml) water

Make into a tea in the usual way, strain, and reduce the liquid to ¼ of a pint. Add an equal part of witch hazel and shake well. Dose 2 tablespoons of the mixture in a douche, once daily. Keep refrigerated.

EMOTIONAL USES

Marigold strengthens the emotions in times of crisis, trauma and shock. It helps the person to ground themselves, to take the strength to deal with the crisis. It brings some light and hope in dark times.

Melissa — *Melissa officinalis*

PART USED:	leaves and flowers
PICKING TIME:	June–September
MAIN ACTIONS:	relaxant, digestive
CONSTITUENTS:	volatile oil
COMMON NAMES:	balm, sweet balm, lemon balm

PHYSICAL USES

Soothing and calming, melissa is an excellent remedy for women at the change of life. It regulates and balances the menstrual cycle, reduces hot flushes and night sweats and stops palpitations. It balances the nervous system and can therefore be used for both depression and anxiety: it lifts the spirits in depression and at the same time calms and soothes them in anxiety. Use for insomnia, headache, panic attacks, and dizziness. In PMT melissa is calming and centring, and helps to soothe jangled nerves. It is a heart remedy, so it is used to lower blood pressure, calm the heart and improve the circulation. It is an excellent remedy for the digestion. Melissa can be used as a first-aid remedy for menstrual cramps.

Recipe for palpitations and flushes

Equal parts of melissa
               hawthorn
               motherwort

Make up as a tea (½ oz mixed herbs to 1 pint water) or tincture and take twice daily for 3-4 weeks.

EMOTIONAL USES

I have used melissa a lot for women who have had some kind of sexual trauma, after abortion, rape, surgery, investigative tests, ectopic pregnancy, IUD insertion or extraction, incest or traumatic childbirth. It seems to build or rebuild a sense of identity, to heal the psychic and emotional wounds, and to allow the rage and pain to be expressed and some healing or resolution to take place. Warming and enfolding, melissa helps to unfreeze the frozen places and allow warmth to come in and the beginnings of trust to emerge.

Motherwort

Leonoris cardiaca

PART USED: leaves and flowers
PICKING TIME: June–September
MAIN ACTIONS: cardiac tonic, sedative, gynaecological tonic
CONSTITUENTS: bitter principle, alkaloid, tannin, volatile oil
COMMON NAMES: lion's tail

PHYSICAL USES

Motherwort is an excellent remedy to bring on a delayed period, where there is bloating and a feeling of congestion and pressure. Especially if this is due to tension and irritability. It relaxes muscle spasm and so is used for painful periods. Motherwort is a specific for the menopause and is used for hot flushes and vaginal dryness. A cardiac remedy, it is used for hypertension and palpitations; it helps to regulate the circulation where there are cold extremities. Use for insomnia, anxiety attacks, tension headaches and dizziness.

EMOTIONAL USES

Motherwort is for mothers, biological or otherwise – those of us who give, sacrifice and patiently watch our children or our projects grow. It is calming and open-hearted, both qualities we need in abundance when mothering. Hope and patience do not go amiss either, but centring and the right use of energy are paramount.

Mugwort

Artemisia vulgaris

PART USED: stem, leaves and flowers
PICKING TIME: June–August
MAIN ACTIONS: relaxant, astringent, digestive, antiseptic
CONSTITUENTS: volatile oils, tannin, bitters

PHYSICAL USES

Mugwort is a relaxing gynaecological tonic which is especially suitable for girls at puberty. It is relaxing, so that it helps to ease the muscle tension that causes period pains, and is also astringent, helping to reduce excess blood loss and to dry up discharges. It is a tonic and will regulate the menstrual cycle, and brings on delayed periods due to stress, helping the blood to flow freely. Mugwort is an antiseptic and so is useful for womb infections such as PID, chronic thrush or cystitis, to build up the immune system and make the body resistant to disease. It is a liver remedy and is helpful in PMT. Used together with antibiotic therapy for the treatment of venereal disease, mugwort can help to minimize the suppressant effect of these drugs and thus possible after-effects.

To bring on a delayed period

1 oz (25g) mugwort
1 oz (25g) pennyroyal
2 pints (1 litre) water

Mix the ingredients and slowly bring to the boil. Simmer for 15 minutes and then strain. Take during the course of the day.

EMOTIONAL USES

Mugwort is used for clarity when there is confusion, indecision and uncertainty; for people who find it hard to make decisions and choices. It calms the mind, clears the head and allows for a clearer vision. Mugwort opens up possibilities for those who lack vision and strengthens the will for people who feel powerless or impotent. It counters negativity, depression and feelings of hopelessness by enabling women to connect with their inner strength and wisdom.

Myrrh

PART USED:	resin
MAIN ACTIONS:	antiseptic, anti-microbial, anti-catarrhal, emmenagogic
COMMON NAMES:	didthin, bowl

PHYSICAL USES

Myrrh stimulates the immune system and the white blood cell count. It is an excellent remedy whenever there is infection. Use for PID, chronic thrush, trichamoniasis and herpes. As a powerful astringent it is useful for fibroids and endometriosis. Myrrh will staunch heavy bleeding and clear up discharges. A tonic to the lining of the vagina and uterus, it can be used for vaginal dryness and fibroids. It can help to bring on menstruation when the cycle is irregular or the period is delayed. Myrrh is helpful in cases of stubborn cystitis.

Note: Myrrh is a strong remedy, and should not be used for more than three weeks at a stretch. If you need to repeat the treatment wait three weeks before taking it again.

EMOTIONAL USES

Use myrrh for emotional clarity when there is confusion and uncertainty. It will help to clear the low clouds blocking the sun. Myrrh works on the will, on that part of our mind which can design and create our present and future realities. The mind is a powerful tool and as yet we only use a small part of it. The power to visualize is one of the first tools to be developed in order to give the will control over our lives. We visualize all the time, unconsciously, and these images have a powerful effect on our lives. If we imagine disaster long enough and in enough detail, disaster will oblige us by appearing. Conversely, if we imagine good fortune it tends to manifest itself. This, I feel is the basis for 'luck': an inner alignment, a fixed focus which is open enough and flexible enough to catch everyday happenings and turn them to our advantage, by being intuitive enough to recognize hunches and bold enough to act on them.

Nettle

Urtica dioica

PART USED:	leaves, stem and flowers
PICKING TIME:	May–September
MAIN ACTIONS:	astringent, anti-haemorrhagic, mineralizer, diuretic
CONSTITUENTS:	tannin, iron, vitamin C, histamine
COMMON NAMES:	noedl (Anglo-Saxon for needle)

PHYSICAL USES

Nettle is a strong astringent and so is used for blood loss anywhere in the body, but particularly from the uterus and bladder. Use in the menopause if there is flooding and a shortened cycle. Nettle contains iron and so is the treatment of choice for anaemia and low blood pressure. It is a strong diuretic, and can be used to lower blood pressure and to reduce water retention. It is used in cystitis to soothe the inflamed tissue, stop any bleeding and generally act as a tonic to the whole area. As an astringent nettle can also be helpful for fibroids and endometriosis. Finally, nettle is a powerful blood cleanser and is used for the skin in eczema, acne, urticaria and boils.

EMOTIONAL USES

Nettle is a fire herb and as such it helps women to contact that element within themselves. When a person feels like a victim, overwhelmed by feelings, depressed, passive and over-sensitive, nettle will help her to contact the warrior within. It is for women who are warriors, who fight battles on behalf of the less able, and who at times feel defeated or burnt out.

Pennyroyal

Mentha pugelium

PART USED:	stem, leaves and flowers
PICKING TIME:	July and August
MAIN ACTIONS:	emmenagogic, astringent, gynaecological tonic
CONSTITUENTS:	volatile oil
COMMON NAMES:	pudding grass, lurk-in-the-ditch, run-by-the-ground

PHYSICAL USES

Pennyroyal is a powerful emmenagogue and will bring on even the most stubbornly delayed period; for this reason, it should not be taken during pregnancy as it will harm the foetus and probably cause a miscarriage. It can be used for menstrual cramps where the circulation is sluggish and there is congestion in the womb. It will increase the menstrual flow for women whose loss is slight. It is a strong antiseptic and can be used in infections like PID.

EMOTIONAL USES

Working as powerfully as it does on the womb, pennyroyal has a centring and strengthening action. The womb can be called the centre of our will (the lower will, if you like). It is the *hara*, the centre of balance, the place we move out from. Pennyroyal can help to rebuild this centre of energy, when a woman feels she has lost a sense of herself, through trauma, sickness or repeated childbirth, and needs to reconnect with this primal energy source.

Poke Root

Phytolacca americana

PART USED:	root
PICKING TIME:	late autumn or early spring
MAIN ACTIONS:	lymphatic remedy, anti-rheumatic, detoxifying
CONSTITUENTS:	saponins, alkaloids, resins, tannin

PHYSICAL USES

A deep-acting blood cleanser, poke root is the remedy of choice for any infection, such as PID or chronic thrush, for swollen breasts, breast lumps and mastitis. Use it for a short period (10-15 days) after an infection to cleanse the system; it is also helpful in the treatment of herpes.

Caution: in large doses, poke root is a powerful emetic and purgative. DO NOT TAKE DURING PREGNANCY.

As a blood cleanser

Five drops of the tincture three times daily.

EMOTIONAL USES

This is a powerful cleansing herb, both for the emotions and for the body. It is to be used with care when there are powerful and destructive emotions, for example, jealousy, which can be overwhelming in its intensity and force, greed, anger, envy, rage; all the very bitterest of feelings, long-held resentments, old emotional patterns. Poke root is also helpful for the long term treatment of addictions to alcohol, tobacco, food, and to a lesser extent, drugs. It helps to cleanse the body and release the powerful emotions the addict is trying to suppress with the drug. Take 2-3 drops of the tincture every three hours in acute addictive phases, and the normal dose otherwise.

Raspberry Leaf

Rubus idaeus

PART USED: leaves and fruit
PICKING TIME: throughout the growing season
MAIN ACTIONS: astringent, tonic
CONSTITUENTS: volatile oil, pectin

PHYSICAL USES

This is an excellent remedy for the pregnant woman. It strengthens the uterus, eases childbirth, prevents miscarriage and promotes breastfeeding. Drink after the first 12 weeks of pregnancy and throughout labour. It is also useful for discharges, heavy periods and painful periods. Take 1 teaspoon (2.5g) of the dried herb in a cup of boiling water.

EMOTIONAL USES

A gentle emotional relaxant for fearful mothers, for women pregnant for the first time who are over-anxious. It is calming, soothing and gently relaxing. It helps to build up nervous tissue, giving the woman the necessary endurance for the work that lies ahead. Take the tea 2-3 times daily.

Red Clover

Trifolium praetense

PART USED:	flowers
PICKING TIME:	May–July
MAIN ACTIONS:	blood cleanser, relaxant, gynaecological remedy
CONSTITUENTS:	flavonoids, oestrogenic substances, coumarins
COMMON NAMES:	trefoil, purple clover

PHYSICAL USES

Clover is deep-acting and very powerful. It is used mainly for chronic, serious conditions, which is why it has the reputation for being a remedy against cancer and other growths. Use in endometriosis, fibroids, PID and chronic herpes. It is an astringent and so it is helpful in heavy periods. The tea has been used in local infections, thrush and trichamoniasis, as a douche. It is also a liver remedy and so can help to increase absorption and stimulate digestion. Red clover is a skin remedy to be used in chronic, persistent conditions like eczema and acne. It has a relaxant action and is useful for anxiety and tension associated with chronic illness.

EMOTIONAL USES

Again, this is a deeply penetrating remedy which can draw out long-buried emotions, old hurts, and powerful feelings. As such it needs to be used with care. But where there is a serious and potentially life-threatening illness, urgent action has to be taken to get to the bottom of the problem. For any chronic illness to have developed, many years will have gone into creating the conditions for this to be possible. Buried resentments, unexpressed anger and old wounds can all accumulate and, if not expressed emotionally, will tend to affect the physical body. This is not to say that the illness is a punishment, as some alternative practitioners seem to think: merely for 'dis-ease' to occur there must be a fundamental imbalance in the energies of the body. Which is why visualization techniques work so well in the treatment of cancer: they are able to penetrate into deep layers of the subconscious, places to which we usually don't have access. Red clover is a remedy for the times when it feels as if there is no hope, for desperation and despair.

Rosemary   *Rosmarinus officinalis*

PART USED: flowers, leaves and stem
PICKING TIME: May–September
MAIN ACTIONS: stimulant, digestive, antiseptic
CONSTITUENTS: volatile oil, tannin, resin, camphor
COMMON NAMES: polar plant, compass weed, incensier,
                  romero

PHYSICAL USES

Rosemary is a circulatory stimulant. It increases the rate at which
blood flows around the body, generally improves the circulation
and therefore the well-being of every part. Use for people with
poor circulation, cold hands and feet, low blood pressure,
dizziness, weakness and exhaustion. Rosemary especially
stimulates the blood flow to the brain and is an excellent remedy
for migraine, depression, poor concentration and bad memory. It
improves the circulation to the reproductive organs and so is
helpful for period pains caused by cold, congestion or lack of
muscle tone. Rosemary is traditionally used as a treatment and
preventative for hardening of the arteries.

EMOTIONAL USES

As a heart remedy, Rosemary is concerned with the expression
of emotions, particularly love. It helps to open the heart, allowing
the free flow of these energies and at the same time, encourages
discrimination in the use of open-heartedness. Some women are
too open and too willing to take on the pain and suffering of others.
They lack discrimination and don't know how to regulate the

expression of these energies. These people get burnt out easily, that is to say, they are drained and exhausted by the impossible task they have set themselves. They need to have stronger boundaries and practise more self protection if they are going to be able to give the way they want.

Sage

Salvia officinalis

PART USED:	leaves, stem and flowers
PICKING TIME:	July
MAIN ACTIONS:	astringent, haemostatic, diuretic, antiseptic
CONSTITUENTS:	volatile oil, tannin, resins
COMMON NAMES:	sawge (Anglo-Saxon), from Latin *Salvere* (to be well)

PHYSICAL USES

Sage is a hormonal balancer and is particularly useful during the menopause to stop excess blood loss, hot flushes and sensitivity to temperature changes. Sage is very drying and some women have found that it dries out their skin: if this is the case, add marigold to the mixture to balance things out. As an astringent, sage is useful in the treatment of fibroids and endometriosis. It will also help to regulate irregular cycles in puberty. Taken hot as a tea, sage will bring on a period, and therefore it is not recommended during pregnancy.

It is a mood-elevating plant for debility, exhaustion and any physical condition which has its roots in anxiety or worry. Sage is a diuretic and so is useful for water retention, sluggish kidneys, cystitis and kidney stones. It is an important remedy to regulate blood sugar levels, whether they are high or low, but insulin-dependent diabetics should be under the care of a herbalist so as not to upset the equilibrium they have obtained.

Douche for thrush and leucorrhoea

3 fl oz (80ml) rose water
⅓ fl oz (10ml) tincture of sage
⅓ fl oz (10ml) tincture of archangel

Mix and use one tablespoon of the mixture diluted in ½ pint (250ml) of warm water; use daily.

EMOTIONAL USES

Sage is concerned with expression. We express ourselves in a variety of ways, through our spoken language and through the creative acts we perform. Sage is useful for those with blocks to their creativity, performers, artists, writers or musicians who have become stuck, who are looking for new ideas, new directions; also for those who have yet to find a creative outlet, a means of expressing themselves. Sage is also indicated for those who have problems with speech, stutters, poor memory, or shyness: it helps the free flow of energy through the throat and frees the emotional charge behind these problems in communication.

Shepherd's Purse

Capsella bursa pastoris

PART USED: leaves, stem and flowers
PICKING TIME: June–September
MAIN ACTIONS: astringent, anti-haemorrhagic
CONSTITUENTS: organic acid, tannin, alkaloid, volatile oil, resin
COMMON NAMES: witches' pouches, Diana's arrow, rattle pouches, pick purse, mother's heart

PHYSICAL USES

A powerful astringent, shepherd's purse is used in the treatment of heavy periods, particularly at the menopause; fibroids, endometriosis and vaginal discharges. It is a kidney remedy, used for cystitis or kidney stones, and a mild diuretic. Use in thrush, where there is a lot of heat and inflammation; shepherd's purse is cooling and soothing.

EMOTIONAL USES

Shepherd's purse helps to develop the will and so is indicated for people who are easily swayed by others, who lose sight of what their desires are and become overwhelmed by those of others. It helps to ground people and make them more stable, less easily influenced, more self-assured. For people with low self-esteem who don't feel entitled to have their own opinions, space or time.

Skullcap

Scutelaria laterifolia

PART USED:	aerial parts
PICKING TIME:	August and September
MAIN ACTIONS:	bitter, astringent, nerve tonic, relaxant
CONSTITUENTS:	essential oil, tannins, bitters, iron salts, calcium, potassium, magnesium, flavonoid glycosides

PHYSICAL USES

Skullcap is an excellent remedy for nervous tension and physical and mental exhaustion, and is relaxing and restorative to the entire nervous system. It is used to relieve painful periods and pre-menstrual tension. It is also a remedy for high blood pressure, palpitations and heart pain. Take before bed for insomnia. It is used for menopausal depression and anxiety symptoms as well as for hot flushes. It helps to regulate the menstrual cycle.
   DO NOT TAKE IN PREGNANCY.

For period pain

¼ oz (7g) skullcap
¼ oz (7g) cramp bark

Mix and make into a tea in the normal way. Sip throughout the course of the day.

EMOTIONAL USES

Skullcap is useful where there has been a great shock or fright, for what I call frozen panic, where the person has palpitations, shivering and sweating. It can be used in the treatment of nightmares for children and adults alike. For acute weight loss due to anxiety, a loss of the will to live, despair, disappointment, death of loved ones, stillbirth, miscarriage or abortion. It helps the grieving process along, especially if the death was some time ago and the person has not allowed herself to grieve fully.

For insomnia due to fear or grief and for nightmares, drink 1 cupful (1 teaspoon (2.5g) in 1 cup of boiling water) before retiring. Skullcap is also drunk at funerals for the same purpose.

Squaw Vine

Mitchella repens

PART USED:	aerial parts
PICKING TIME:	between April and June
MAIN ACTIONS:	astringent, reproductive tonic, diuretic
CONSTITUENTS:	mucilage, saponins

PHYSICAL USES

Squaw vine is an excellent remedy for painful periods, especially when they come early and there is heavy bleeding. It is used for fibroids as a long-term treatment. Taken during the last month of pregnancy, it helps to ease labour and promotes contractions. It is a remedy for cystitis and vaginal discharge. It can be used for threatened miscarriage.

To prepare for childbirth

Mix with raspberry leaf
1 teaspoon (2.5g) of each herb in 2 cups of boiling water. Leave to infuse for 10-15 minutes. Take twice daily.

EMOTIONAL USES

For mental exhaustion, feelings of being overburdened and being unable to cope, because of taking on too many responsibilities. It helps to change the mental attitude, to make the person feel less responsible for everything. For the initial shock of new motherhood, for the mothers of twins and triplets, for post-natal depression when the woman feels that she cannot cope. For tearfulness, helplessness and exhaustion. Take in the usual manner.

St John's Wort

Hypericum perfoliatum

PART USED: leaves, flowers and stem

PICKING TIME: around midsummer

MAIN ACTIONS: anti-inflammatory, astringent, analgesic, sedative

CONSTITUENTS: glycosides, rutin, volatile oil, tannin, resin, pectin

COMMON NAMES: *fuga daemonum* (Latin), in reference to its power to banish evil spirits

PHYSICAL USES

One of the main herbs used for the menopause. It is excellent for hot flushes and sweating. Its main action is on the nervous system – calming, restorative, energizing but not stimulating. Use for anxiety, mild depression, insomnia, nightmares. It is also useful for sciatica, neuralgia and painful periods. Sage can be added to mixtures for PID, fibroids and endometriosis as a pain-killer. It acts as an astringent for bleeding from the kidneys and the womb. Note: people with severe or long-standing depression should not take this plant, nor should those who suffer from photosensitivity, as it will aggravate both conditions.

EMOTIONAL USES

St John's wort is used for women who have lost their direction in life, who need to contact their inner selves, who want to reorientate. It is especially useful for strong, capable people, who for various reasons have lost sight of themselves and need help to find their road again. For this reason, St John's wort is particularly useful during the change of life. Often at this age women can undergo a crisis of meaning. At a time when they are again faced with themselves after many years of mothering and living with that identity, they have to recreate their lives. Now they have the luxury of time and space to themselves, but it can come as a shock, and many women feel disorientated at their new-found freedom. St John's wort can help in this reorienting process.

Vitex

Vitex agnus castus

PART USED:	seeds
PICKING TIME:	autumn
MAIN ACTIONS:	hormonal balancer
CONSTITUENTS:	hormone type substances
COMMON NAME:	monk's pepper

PHYSICAL USES

Vitex is believed to act on the pituitary gland regulating the secretion of progesterone. For this reason it is the remedy for PMT; taken for two months, it will right even the most stubborn cases. It will also treat acne associated with hormone imbalance, thrush due to the same cause, chronic painful periods and severe heavy bleeding. It is a treatment for pre-menstrual migraine and depression, and is helpful to regulate the menstrual cycle after a woman has come off the contraceptive pill. For menopausal symptoms which are severe, vitex is also useful. Progesterone is said to block the development of endometriosis and therefore vitex is indicated in the treatment of that condition. Fibroids respond well to vitex taken over the course of several months.

How to take Vitex

Vitex works best as a tincture; you can make your own or buy it ready-made. I have never used tablets so cannot pass an opinion on them. Take it first thing in the morning: this is when the pituitary is most active and thus most susceptable to treatment. Take 15 drops once only, in the morning. You need to take it for at least two menstrual cycles to see a change. Some women have reported that in the first month their symptoms were slightly worse:

if this happens, persist, and next month they will be much better. After your symptoms have gone, gradually cut down the dosage. It is important to do this slowly, month by month, so that your body will have time to adjust and will continue to stay well.

EMOTIONAL USES

Vitex is for women. It is a celebration of ourselves, our cycles, our bodies, our creativity and our lives. Vitex helps women who have lost this whole vision, women over-identified with the intellectual or with the emotional side of the personality. It is a balancing remedy; neither one aspect nor another should be in excess.

Wild Yam

Dioscorea villosa

PART USED: dried root
PICKING TIME: autumn
MAIN ACTIONS: relaxant, astringent, anti-inflammatory,
                  digestive
CONSTITUENTS: steroidal saponins, alkaloids, tannin

PHYSICAL USES

This herb was once the main source of the hormones used in the manufacture of the contraceptive pill. It is used for pain anywhere in the reproductive system: painful periods, ovarian pain, pain during labour and post partum. It is a digestive tonic, used for the gall bladder in gallstones, stomach cramps, colitis, colic and nausea. Its steroid content makes it useful for treating rheumatism and arthritis as well as eczema and dermatitis. It has been used with success in the treatment of threatened miscarriage; take 30 drops every 30-60 minutes.

AVOID IN PREGNANCY, EXCEPT FOR THREATENED MISCARRIAGE.

EMOTIONAL USES

For infertility due to worry or over-preoccupation with having a child, especially for women over 35. It is centring, calming, grounding and stabilizing. Use to treat sexual trauma, confusion over one's sexual identity and the fear of sexual maturity. It is an excellent remedy for adolescents when they are experimenting and questioning their sexual identity. It is also a useful remedy for women at the menopause and afterwards, when again, women often re-evaluate their sexual needs.

Yarrow   *Achillea millefolium*

PART USED: flowers, leaves and stem
PICKING TIME: June–September
MAIN ACTIONS: emmenagogic, haemostatic, sedative,
                 diaphoretic, asatringent, tonic, bitter
CONSTITUENTS: bitter principles, volatile oil, tannin,
                 potassium
COMMON NAME: gerwe (Anglo-Saxon), devil's nettle,
                 devil's plaything, herbe militaire

PHYSICAL USES

Yarrow is an excellent first-aid remedy for menstrual cramps due
to weakness and cold, taken hot as a tea and sweetened with honey.
It can treat excess menstrual flow in the same way. It is useful in
the menopause where there is flooding, similarly in puberty. Its
astringent qualities are helpful in treating fibroids. Yarrow can be
used to treat non-infectious vaginal discharges. Taken for long
periods, yarrow will help relieve tension in the pelvis. It stops
haemorrhages and so is useful for nosebleeds, blood in the urine
and other bloody discharges. It is used in the treatment of
thrombosis and varicose veins, and any disease of the circulation;
coronary disease (when mixed with hawthorn), and Reynaud's
disease. It has a normalizing effect on the heart muscle, making
it beat more regularly and strongly. It is also sedative, lowering
high blood pressure caused by stress and anxiety; it is a bitter
tonic to the digestive system and hence it is used to increase
absorption. It is a urinary antiseptic when combined with other
herbs for recurrent cystitis and the symptomatic relief of PMT.

Tea for menstrual cramps

Equal parts of the following (½ oz (12.5g) in total)
yarrow
motherwort
sage (if the bleeding is very heavy)

Add to 1 pint (500ml) of water. Stand for 10 minutes covered, mix with honey and drink during the day.

EMOTIONAL USES

Yarrow is another warrior herb. For the fighters, those women who are defenders of the weak, the needy, the helpless, who want to fight institutions, patriarchal structures, injustice wherever it occurs. It is also for those fighting internal battles against addictions, mental illness, depression and fear. Yarrow strengthens and solidifies, and gives courage and energy to continue struggling.

Glossary

CONSTITUENTS

Alkaloids: These are the strongest and the largest group of plant constituents and many modern drugs are derived from plant alkaloids. Examples include morphine, dopamine and mescaline. Their actions vary widely and so they cannot be described generally.

Allantoin: Found in the flowers and leaves of comfrey, this substance enters the skin easily and heals bones, muscles and ligaments.

Bioflavonoids: Or vitamin P, found in berries and citrus fruits. It strengthens the blood vessels, makes them more flexible and resilient, protects against haemorrhage and aids the absorption of vitamin C.

Bitters: These are a group of substances widely distributed in plants. They have a bitter taste, hence their name. They stimulate the liver, increase the secretion of bile and thus stimulate digestion of food, absorption and the numerous other functions the liver has. They work by reflex action from the mouth, via the taste buds, and for this reason they should not be sweetened.

Vitamin B12: Found in comfrey, B12 is needed for the absorption of iron into the body. Some sources claim that vegans and vegetarians need extra B12 in their diets, others claim that they are able to manufacture this.

Coumarins: They are believed to have an anti-clotting action on the blood.

Flavonoids: Very common, they have several actions, such as assisting the circulation, and acting as antispasmodics, diuretics and heart stimulants.

Glycosides: Some are heart remedies, others are bitters working on the liver.

Gums and Mucilages: These are both protective; they cover tissues with a layer of gummy material which aids healing. They are used where there is inflammation, especially for the lungs, kidneys and bladder. They are destroyed by heat, so remedies containing mucilage, when this action is required, should be taken in cold infusions (left overnight in cold water).

Histamine: It is used to counter allergic actions in the body.

Inulin: A type of fruit sugar.

Resin: A solid often found with volatile oils e.g. pine resin.

Rutin: Has an action very similar to that of bioflavonoids.

Salicyclic acid: It is a pain killer which lowers fever; it is anti-inflammatory and a sedative and kidney remedy.

Saponins: These appear to be similar to hormones and many saponin-containing plants do act on the gynaecological system, backing up this theory. They also work on the lungs as expectorants. They aid digestion and the absorption of food.

Silica: Found in all grasses, silica is a wound healer and a soothing remedy for inflammation, used especially for the lungs and kidneys.

Sucrose: A type of sugar.

Tannins: These are astringent in that they reduce the water content of the body and stop discharges and haemorrhages. They can affect protein absorption into the body and therefore plants high in tannin should only be taken for a short time, such as myrrh.

Valerianic acids: Sedative in action.

Volatile oils: These give plants their scent, and as their name suggests, they are dissolved in boiling water. For this reason herbal teas made with boiling water are often more effective than tinctures and tablets. Volatile oils are antiseptic, generally relaxant and stimulate the digestion.

ACTIONS

Analgesic: pain-killing.

Antiviral/microbial: kills viruses and bacteria, or reduces their virulency.

Antiseptic: kills bacteria.

Antihaemorrhagic: stops bleeding.

Anticatarrhal: reduces catarrh.

Antispasmodic: muscle relaxant, reduces pain due to muscle spasm.

Astringent: dries up haemorrhages and discharges, strengthens tissues generally, heals wounds.

Blood cleanser/purifier: encourages the excretion of waste products via the blood and kidneys.

Carminative: reduces wind or flatulence.

Cholagogue, cholagogic: increases the flow of bile from the gall bladder and hence liver function.

Demulcent: soothing to inflamed tissues.

Digestive or digestive stimulant: increases secretion of digestive enzymes and so aids absorption and digestion of food.

Diaphoretic: causes sweating.

Diuretic: increases urine production and secretion.

Expectorant: expels mucus from the lungs and respiratory tract.

Emmenagogue, emmenagogic: brings on a delayed period, causes abortion.

Haemostatic: stops bleeding.

Healing: aids tissues to heal themselves.

Hepatic: stimulates the action of the liver and regulates its function.

Hypertensive: raises blood pressure.

Hypotensive: lowers blood pressure.

Mineralizer: increases the mineral content of the bloodstream.

Nutritive: has properties which are nutritious to body generally.

Sedative: causes relaxation and drowsiness.

Systemic: a remedy which affects the whole body.

Tonic: a general term which in herbal lore means anything which balances and regulates the function of an organ or system, e.g. a circulatory tonic regulates the circulation and heart.

Index

Note: individual herbs are listed alphabetically in the Herbal, pages 89-152